T0356982

A Straightforward Guide for
Every Woman at Every Stage of Life

THE HORMONE

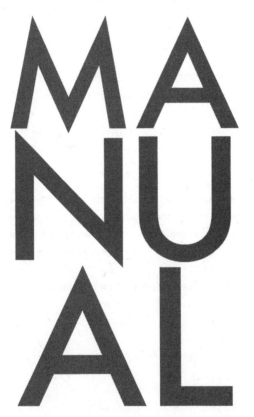

MANUAL

JULIE TAYLOR MD MPH

RESOLVE
EDITIONS

Published by Resolve Editions, an imprint of
Forefront Books, Nashville, Tennessee.
Distributed by Simon & Schuster.

Library of Congress Control Number: 2025901779

Print ISBN: 978-1-63763-343-4
E-book ISBN: 978-1-63763-344-1

Cover Design by Bruce Gore, Gore Studio, Inc.
Interior Design by Mary Susan Oleson, Blu Design Concepts

Printed in the United States of America

This book is dedicated to my incredible children, William, Gemma, and Wyatt, whom I love and adore with every ounce of who I am. And to my loving and devoted husband, Drew. Everything I do is for all of you. To my parents, who have supported me from day one, thank you for all you are and all you do. I am indebted to you. To my brother, who lifted me up as a young girl and believed in me. To my grandfather, who from a young age instilled in me the value of education. And to my patients, who have taught me all I know. You have fulfilled me in ways I cannot express. Thank you for entrusting me to care for you. In turn, you have given me purpose and given me the wings to continue to help more and more people. And to God, who makes all things possible. You have grounded me, guided me, and given me wisdom and clarity along this incredible journey.

Contents

AUTHOR'S NOTE

When you stop and think about the incredible industrial and technological advances our society has achieved throughout history, the list is nothing short of astounding. Imagine the trial and error, the failed attempts, and the lessons learned during all that innovation. Over time, people have documented what works and what doesn't, and the details of how they approached their new inventions. These documents are called "manuals." You surely have plenty of them, whether they're for your computer or your refrigerator, your washing machine or your car. Companies have manuals for their business policies, and to document the processes of manufacturing their products. Why? You wouldn't build a skyscraper hundreds of feet high without documenting the process so you can repeat the effort. Why design an electric self-driving car if you can't build a fleet of them? We, as humans, don't want to achieve something just once—we want to create the how-to guide, and then constantly revise and improve upon it.

For instance, in order to fly an airplane full of people from Los Angeles to New York City, there is a preflight checklist—specific steps the pilots and flight crews must take in order to ensure a safe journey for all aboard. Of course, there are unexpected events, but there are also steps to be taken should those occur. There are even backup plans for the backup plans. Certain inarguable laws of physics are at play when it comes to flying an airplane, and experts work within those laws to create manuals to operate the plane.

Wouldn't it be incredible if we had a specific check-list to follow when it comes to our own bodies? While we are not airplanes, there are things we experience that have happened to our ancestors and will happen to future generations. There are some distinct truths that apply to us all. You'd think by now there would be a clear-cut list of instructions for how to successfully, safely, and healthfully operate our own bodies, wouldn't you?

We are, in fact, the most powerful and most awesome piece of machinery ever designed. The human body is incredible, and while there are certainly some of its functions that are not fully understood, we have amassed a vast amount of knowledge about it. That knowledge, if used correctly, can help us. Immensely.

But there's a problem.

That knowledge hasn't been made available to you in a way that you can easily apply to your life. Instead, tracking down information about how to make your body function at peak performance can feel like a wild-goose chase. There may be times when you sit in the doctor's office and feel you are the only one who has ever gone through what you are going through. Do you agree?

There are a myriad of reasons why this is the case, and part of the problem is that as a medical society, we have moved away from looking at the whole patient. Think about it; there used to be a time when doctors made house calls and spent the necessary time getting to know their patients. There wasn't an array of specialists for every organ of the body. You had one doctor who put all the pieces together.

You didn't go to one doctor who then referred you to another doctor and another doctor. But now, patients are often left frustrated and dissatisfied and wonder how anyone will ever solve their symptoms. We have moved away from focusing on the whole patient and instead have moved in the direction of monetizing medicine and overregulating doctors. Anytime money enters the picture, the situation changes.

Turn on the television at any hour of the day and, within a matter of minutes, you're likely to see a commercial for a prescription drug. Many of them have done wonders for helping us live longer lives, such as insulin for type 1 diabetes or antibiotics for severe bacterial infections. But what happens when doctors are afforded an easy "fix" to help their patients feel better with a pill rather than getting to the root of the issue? Patients want a quick fix. Doctors want to keep their patients, so they whip out their prescription pads and prescribe medications for a temporary solution rather than assessing their patients' overall needs.

I'm not here, however, to dissect or investigate the methods or motivations of Western medicine.

The fact remains that the information you need to solve your health challenges and begin living a life defined by vitality and optimal health hasn't been made readily available to you. Why shouldn't you have an easy way to understand what is happening to your body and identify ways to fix it? Most of the patients who walk through my office door are searching for just that. And I would hedge a bet that maybe you are too.

The bottom line is this: No one is looking out for your health and well-being more than you are. Not your doctor. Certainly not the pharmaceutical companies or the food conglomerates. Not the actors on the commercials selling you another quick fix. The buck stops with you. Your body is your plane, and you are the pilot.

What I aim to do is give *you* the manual.

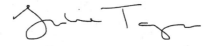

Chapter 1

MY JOURNEY INTO
FUNCTIONAL MEDICINE

I never heard the terms "functional medicine" or "preventive medicine" when I was in medical school. Did you know that preventive medicine is one of the recognized residencies that medical students can pursue after medical school, but it is rarely—if ever—presented to medical students? Why is that? There are several prestigious institutions around the country that have preventive medicine residency programs, but medical students often don't hear about them. It was by accident that I even heard about preventive and functional medicine, but here's how I discovered what ended up becoming a very fulfilling career in medicine.

It all started in 2010. I'd finished medical school and moved from Michigan back home to California to begin my primary care residency. But, from day one and to my surprise, I found I was completely miserable. Look, you don't have to tell me that residency isn't supposed to be a cakewalk—I knew that. But this was on another level. My patients were being shoved into a box based on protocols decided by administrators (not doctors), and it all felt like big business that wasn't really benefiting the patient. I grappled with the thought that if this was the way medicine was being practiced, I really didn't want any part of it. I despised every minute of my conventional medicine residency and realized something had to change, and quickly.

A little over a year into my program, I finally reached the point when I needed to walk away. I wasn't sure if I was walking away from medicine as a whole—since I didn't really have a backup plan—but I knew I had to leave what I was currently doing. I really grappled with the thought of leaving medicine, as I had wanted to be a doctor all my life, beginning in elementary school. How could this be the end? What was I going to do now?

Insurance Companies Are Ruining Patients' Health

I need to stop here for a moment and look at conventional medicine as we know it. Like most fields in allopathic medicine, medication is king, insurance companies are dictators, pharmaceutical companies are puppeteers, and doctors are the puppets. In America, doctors are at the behest of Big Pharma and the hospital administrators who tell them what to do. Physicians finish residency and suddenly the ways in which they can treat their patients and what they can prescribe to them is dictated. Even if they believe something should be different, they can't necessarily practice the way they want to if they are within a medical system and take insurance. I once had a patient who asked her doctor about hormone replacement; he said he couldn't prescribe it but wanted to know how she was being treated by me so he could pass it along to his wife, who was suffering from menopausal symptoms.

Consider the patient's perspective; the first question most patients ask a prospective doctor is, "Are you in network?" Many patients aren't able to choose a doctor based on whether he or she is actually a good fit for them, but instead, whether the physician is covered by their insurance. And if the patient's insurance changes, due to a job change, for example, suddenly they have to jump ship to a new doctor that's in their new network. Furthermore, if a certain treatment isn't covered, most doctors will prescribe something that *is* covered, even if it's not as effective. For instance, a doctor might have to prescribe the generic version of a drug instead of the brand name due to high prescription drug costs.

And, putting aside the medication topic for a second, think about all the preventive medical advice that can help a patient: from supplements to acupuncture, lifestyle changes, diet, exercise, and more. But these options aren't typically discussed between doctor and patient because, once again, none of them are covered by insurance. Doctors aren't able to act independently about what is best for their patient; instead, it's all about what the insurance companies instruct them to do. All too often, this means the patient receives subpar care that is anything but personalized—but hey, at least insurance covers it. To me, that's bad medicine. Insurance companies are ruining patients' health. Period.

Let's rewind for a moment. Back in the days before tests and lab markers were available, medical doctors (MDs) sat and listened to their patients. They took the time to truly know their patients—to meet the family, to see where they lived, to understand their true needs and goals. Physicians used their intellect to creatively assess their patients, draw from their medical experience, and make the ultimate decisions for their patients. They didn't answer to an insurance company, or a hospital administration run by a corporate entity. The decision was made by the MD. This makes sense. After all, they were the ones with the medical education and experience to assess and prescribe what was best for their patients. They were the ones who had the passion for medicine and compassion for people, and who strove every day to ensure their patients received the best care possible.

With this deep internal drive to practice medicine in the way I believed best, I knew I had to leave my existing training. So I met with my residency director and soon thereafter left the program.

My decision was also influenced by the fact that during residency I had my first baby. And to leave him every day for a program I didn't believe in made no sense, but it did make my decision to leave that much easier. So in the days that followed, I went on long walks with my baby, pushing the stroller up and down the hills of my neighborhood, pondering my future career and next steps.

A New Concept: Preventive Medicine

During one of those walks, I was talking with a friend who was in medical school at Loma Linda, where we had met during our master's in public health program. She said, "You know, you should really look into the preventive medicine residency here." Preventive medicine residency? Never heard of it. I thought I had been exposed to all the residency options in medical school. How had I missed that one? I was stunned to learn that there was a whole training program devoted to preventing and reversing disease. I certainly never learned about preventing or reversing disease in medical school. I loved the idea and was intrigued from the outset. After all, I already saw things differently; whether it was how to approach my health or my baby's health, it was all about balancing the body, natural is best, medication is the last resort, and less is more. I had always been inclined to look at treating the root cause of a symptom, whether I had a headache and needed to hydrate or hip pain that needed a massage. I loved the idea of preventive medicine. It was right up my alley.

So I did my research and contacted the residency director the next day. That was in February, and thanks to a position that opened up unexpectedly, by May I had been accepted into the program and started that July.

As I had anticipated, the program was the opposite of my previous residency. From day one, I knew I was right where I was supposed to be. I had to commute an hour each way to the hospital because of where my husband and I were living and the location of his job, but my interest in the program and in creating a career in this type of medicine was worth every minute on the road. I began to learn from physicians who had devoted their careers to preventing and reversing disease, and finally, since graduating from medical school, my medical career was starting to make sense. For the first time, I learned how to take patients off medications and reverse their chronic diseases. I read published studies and analyzed data that showed that patients don't actually need to be on medication for life. I learned how they could take back their health, even if it had declined severely. It was revolutionary!

One of my favorite subjects was hormone replacement therapy and how hormonal imbalance can cause major health issues, including mental health decline. I had a brilliant mentor—a retired surgeon—who ran a clinic where he prescribed bioidentical hormones to men and women. Even though it was my first time encountering this type of practice, I knew instantly that what he was doing made sense. His patients were feeling balanced when they never had before. They had energy. They'd gotten off their medications. It was the type of specialty I knew I loved but never knew existed.

The more I talked about the field of hormones among friends and family, the more I realized that everyone had a hormone story. Whether it was about themselves, their sister, mother, wife—it was unanimous. Everyone had a story. Hormones were an issue everyone dealt with; they just weren't being treated in the way I was discovering. This discovery reignited a passion I had always had for women's health, so I knew I had found the perfect fit. I had contemplated obstetrics-gynecology (OB/Gyn) in medical school but had resisted the lifestyle of long and erratic hours—especially since I wanted to have a family of my own and work-life balance was extremely important to me. To discover a field I could practice in that would greatly benefit women and address their issues in a more concrete way than conventional medicine could ever do, all the while giving me the flexibility to raise my family, was the perfect combination. Plus, having worked for a big hospital corporation during the first year of my conventional residency, I knew I wanted to work for myself and make my own decisions in terms of what was best for my patients—not be ruled by Big Pharma or insurance companies.

So, that's the circuitous route by which I arrived at my private practice in Southern California, where I have the privilege of helping patients live their best life.

Think about Hormones First

So, why am I writing this book? I realize there are a lot of fantastic books on hormones, so what makes this one different? This is *your* manual, a guide you can use to understand your hormones today and for the rest of your life. I want hormones to be the first thing you think about when it comes to your physical health. I want hormones to be the first thing you think about when it comes to your mental health. I want hormones to be the first thing that comes to mind when you have symptoms such as anxiety, panic attacks, depression, sleep issues, muscle pain, fatigue, lack of energy, or low sex drive. When your daughter complains of acne, heavy periods, cramps, headaches, depression, or anxiety, I want you to think about hormones.

I want hormones to be the first thing you think about when your husband complains of being tired, unmotivated, depressed, anxious; has a midlife crisis; or—God forbid—wants a divorce. Or *you* want a divorce. I want deficiency of hormones to be your first thought when your seventy-year-old mom complains of memory loss and the family practitioner is concerned about dementia and is sending her to a neurologist for further studies.

I want you to use this book as a reference guide. Pick it up and refer to the chapter that focuses on your concern. No matter what age or stage of life, there is a chapter that addresses the problem. I want you to remember, for anything short of trauma, hormones should be at the very top of your list to consider and address. Yes, that might sound extreme, but I really want you to understand that hormones affect everything, and you need to consider them regularly. Hormones are the reason we feel how we feel, and we act how we act, and they are intricately woven throughout our body. I want you to have that understanding. And that is why I wrote this book.

While you might think your doctor knows everything, you might be surprised to know that most physicians do not learn about hormones in medical school and how they affect every part of the body. I know that sounds strange, but let me explain a little more. Medical school teaches about the menstrual cycle and ovulation. It teaches about rare genetic disorders that can cause hormone imbalance, like growth hormone deficiency causing short stature. They do not teach about the hormones that I am referring to, and how they can cause so many of the symptoms that women seek help for from their doctor.

Let's look at the Women's Health Initiative (WHI) for a minute and how it affected the way doctors prescribe hormones. In the 1990s the National Institute for Health federally funded a study that looked at postmenopausal women taking synthetic hormone replacement. What they found was that the women had an increased risk of strokes, heart attacks, and breast cancer; and, as you can imagine, almost overnight, every woman went off their hormones, and doctors were fearful to continue prescribing them.[1] What the WHI didn't factor in was that the average age of women in the study was sixty-three years old, and that the women were taking synthetic hormones, not bioidentical hormones (more on that later). In 2011, a consensus statement by the International Menopause Society (IMS) regarding hormone therapy stated the following: "The excessive conservatism engendered by the presentation to the media of the first results of the

WHI in 2002 has disadvantaged nearly a decade of women who may have missed the therapeutic window to reduce their future cardiovascular, fracture, and dementia risk."[2] In 2023, an article in the *Journal of Menopause Society* further investigated the WHI study and called into question the results, saying, "A generation of women has been deprived of HT [hormone therapy] largely as a result of this widely publicized misinterpretation of the data. This article attempts to rectify this misunderstanding, with the goal of helping patients and physicians make informed joint decisions about the use of HT."[3]

Despite these findings, I know physicians who feel like they can't prescribe hormones without being concerned that they are causing harm to their patients. When you go to your doctor and expect her to have all the answers and yet she doesn't, it might not be her fault. It's possible she didn't receive the education necessary during her medical training to adequately help you. I know that sounds surprising, but it is true. However, if you, as the patient, understand what doctors are being taught and how highly regulated physicians are by insurance companies and health administrators, you will better understand what mainstream medicine can and cannot do to help you.

Prescriptions Aren't the Answer

Consider your mental health for a second. What will you do when you go to the doctor for a quick five-minute appointment that maybe took two months to get, and you complain of feeling sad, not like yourself, sleeping poorly, and so on, and your doctor says, "Well, why don't you try this medication [your run-of-the-mill antidepressant]? Don't worry, it's a low dose. Then we'll follow up in a month or two and see how you feel." What else are you going to say other than "Okay, Doc"? After all, this is your doctor, someone whom you trust with your health. If he is saying to try a prescription, you're probably going to do it. You aren't presented with other options, so when you consider that the dose is "very low," and the doctor says it's worked for other patients, what do you have to lose? You figure, *I don't have any other options. I feel terrible. My marriage is falling apart, I can't sleep, and I'm completely depressed. I guess I'll try it.* And so it goes. Years of antidepressants, dose changes, new meds.

Does it help? Maybe. But is it the answer? Is it fixing the root cause? For the majority, I would say no.

Let me reiterate the problem: We as physicians receive a certain education in medical school. Why had I never heard of preventive medicine as a medical student? Because I wasn't taught anything about preventing and reversing disease. This is what medical students learn: the anatomy and physiology of the human body, how it breaks down, and how to fix it with medications and procedures. That's what American medical schools teach by and large. And every MD you come across has had the same education because the information provided within allopathic medical schools is highly regulated. So it's really no wonder that patients are taking Big Pharma drugs.

As medical students, finding the root cause of a symptom is not emphasized. But I strongly believe that this is how medicine should be practiced. We physicians should always be seeking to get to the root of the problem, not masking it. We should approach a symptom with the notion that there is something going on in the body that needs to be analyzed and addressed. And we must remember, most importantly, that the body is a system and all its parts work in conjunction with the others; they don't work in isolation. When someone has a rash, we should be looking at what is going on in the gut first. What is the diet like and how is the gut microbiome? But when does that ever happen? In my mind, every primary care physician should be a functional medicine physician, meaning a doctor who looks at the root of the patient's medical concern.

Let's look at "preventive medicine" versus "functional medicine." I've mentioned both of those terms, but what exactly do they mean? Preventive medicine is a recognized—albeit not highly advertised—medical residency classified by the American College of Graduate Medical Education (ACGME). That means that the curriculum is regulated, and there is an exam that residents must take to become board certified. Most doctors who complete a preventive medicine residency go on to work for a public health department since most preventive medicine programs do not have a lot of clinical exposure like my program did. Rather, they focus more on populations and preventing disease on a wider scale.

"Functional medicine" is a relatively new term coined in the 1990s by Dr. Jeffrey Bland, who considered emerging evidence and connected it to clinical medicine to enable providers to move from a drug-based model of fighting disease to a systemic and patient-focused clinical model that would help reverse chronic diseases. It is a curriculum that is taught by doctors to doctors (and other providers) after, or concurrently with, their conventional medical education. Much of what I do in my clinical practice regarding treating hormones, gut health, stress, toxins, and more, I learned outside of medical school.

One of the core factors of functional medicine is hormones. This extends far beyond the physical issues you may face. In fact, many people may not even realize there's a connection between what they're experiencing emotionally (anxiety, depression, migraines, sleep disorders, and so on) and their own biology. With most ailments that patients face, the majority of the time a close examination of hormones is required. Even if your doctor has said your hormone test results are within normal limits, it is important to understand that this may not be exactly true. Unbalanced hormones can cause very slight symptoms or very severe symptoms. Men and women with very severe symptoms are often riddled with anxiety, plunged into the depths of depression, and at times can be suicidal. Have you ever heard that suicidal thoughts can be caused by a hormone imbalance? This is not a common connection, but it is imperative that people make it. I have seen this in my office several times. And every time, it frustrates me to know that people have been suffering without getting proper assessment and care. This may sound wild, but, in many suicide cases, if a person's hormones had been analyzed and treated, they would have felt like a completely different person and potentially lived a very different life.

Let's Get to the Root Cause

The answer can be so simple. Getting to the root cause of a symptom isn't that difficult. It just takes looking at the patient with a different lens. Because I actually have time to sit down with patients, I get to know their situation, and I make a connection. Allopathic doctors are often "allotted" a certain amount of time with patients, and so even if they wanted to sit with them longer, their time is constrained and overseen by powers outside of their control. Their time isn't their own, and they're not even really allowed to think for themselves. If a doctor accepts a certain insurance, they're being paid by that insurance company based on how many patients they see in a day.[4] The medical business is really being run by insurance companies, and it can quickly become a rat race. The result, unfortunately, is dissatisfied doctors and unhappy patients.

I believe that the vast majority of those who choose to attend medical school genuinely want to help others—it starts with their passion for people. But in today's reality, with insurance companies at the helm, doctors' hands are truly tied. Insurance has hijacked the doctor-patient relationship and the way in which doctors are able to care for their patients. You have people running the show who shouldn't be at all; they aren't interested in the human being. They're interested in the bottom line 100 percent of the time. When doctors are in and out with patients so quickly, very little can be accomplished and that personal connection between patient and doctor gets completely lost. But doctors often feel like they have no other option.

Patients are already paying a lot of money for insurance, so the idea of going to a doctor who doesn't accept it is generally out of the question. But the truth is, the standard medical appointment for an insurance-based practice is typically short and usually symptom focused. Doctors who work in this type of insurance-based practice don't have time to search for the root cause. On the other hand, out-of-pocket providers can spend the time they want to and do the tests they feel are most appropriate regardless of what insurance will cover. In my opinion, the health insurance model is broken and isn't acting in the patients' best interest.

You can't really treat a patient when you only see them for a few minutes. But the fact that I don't accept insurance means I'm not beholden to the standard script of insurance companies, which in turn allows me to be a better doctor than I otherwise would have been if I were practicing in a different system. I am able to marry basic science with clinical judgment and consider the body as a whole to determine how best to address my patients' symptoms.

Hormones Are Everything

Hormones really aren't complicated. Surely you have heard someone exclaim, "Oh, she's just hormonal," when a woman responds in a way that seems aggressive or erratic. I was called this by a postmenopausal woman when I was pregnant with my first child. I'll never forget it because it just sounded so weird, especially coming from another (hormonal) woman. It's no wonder the word "hormonal" has a bad connotation. It is almost always used about (and against) women and implies that hormones make people crazy, and nothing can be done about it. None of that is actually true. After all, we all have hormones—both men and women. They make us who we are and without them we would simply be a shell of ourselves.

When patients come into a doctor's office complaining of what they feel are hormone imbalances and they are told that their hormones are normal and there is nothing to be done, they suffer, their families suffer, their children suffer, and society suffers. I don't want families to break apart when they don't need to. I don't want teenagers who are battling a hormone-disordered puberty to suffer, only to be prescribed a lifelong cocktail of medications. I don't want the fifty-year-old menopausal woman to consider suicide because she can't sleep and is severely depressed, and her meds aren't working, and she feels completely hopeless. I don't want the forty-five-year-old man to treat his low testosterone with drugs and alcohol because he has no energy and feels anxious and depressed and doesn't know why, so he searches for ways to suppress the way he feels.

Doctors have been getting it wrong for far too long. It's not their fault though. It's the fault of the educational system and it's time to reeducate the system. It starts with what we learn in medical school, but until we tackle that behemoth, I want you to discover the truth that your hormones might very well be the first place to look no matter what you've got going on medically, emotionally, and physically.

So let's get into it.

Chapter 2

INFANCY AND CHILDHOOD

Welcome to the chapter on Infancy and Childhood. Babies are amazing little beings who rely entirely on their moms for everything during those crucial first days, weeks, and months. Because of this total dependence, I think it's important to first talk about mom's health. How a mom takes care of herself can really set the stage for her baby's development and well-being. So, before we dive into the specifics of infancy and childhood, let's take a moment to focus on the moms. Everything from nutrition and mental health to everyday lifestyle choices plays a huge role in this journey. Keeping moms healthy and happy is key to giving babies the best possible start.

Don't worry, we'll get into much more depth about postpartum matters later in the book.

When I had my first baby, I was in my intern year of training. For a young doctor, this is the year when sleep deprivation and stress are at their highest. I had thirty-hour hospital calls and lots of demands placed on me, but fortunately I was able to maintain a healthy balance outside of work. I focused on exercising regularly—running and practicing yoga a few times a week. I made sure to eat healthy, and my diet consisted primarily of vegetables, fiber, and lean protein. I spent quality time with my husband and got good sleep at every opportunity.

Much of my great experience with my first pregnancy had to do with my wonderful and supersmart Harvard-trained OB/Gyn, Dr. Diana Currie, who was my saving grace. She prepared me for birth and the first few months of life with my baby. I loved how she approached me as a new physician and new mom, and was so good about blending the two. She encouraged a low-key delivery, with the lights off, herbal tea, and relaxing music. I chose to have an epidural so that I could be calm and comfortable, but opted for a very low dose, which still allowed me to feel my contractions and push when I felt them. My son was born within thirty minutes of pushing. It was an incredible experience.

Dr. Currie and I discussed breastfeeding during one of our many prenatal visits as this was very important to me. She warned me that it would hurt until my nipples adjusted and became tough. This discomfort lasted only a couple of weeks, but I am so grateful she gave me a heads-up, because like a lot of mothers, I probably would have felt I was doing something wrong. In fact, a lot of lactation specialists, including the one who consulted with me in the hospital postpartum, say breastfeeding is *not* supposed to hurt. I think this can be very difficult for a mother to hear, especially when it hurts like crazy. If you think about it, the baby is frantically sucking as hard as he can to get the nourishment he needs. And at the same time, the mother's uterus is contracting. It's a cascade of hormone interactions all working together in this very delicate postpartum period. It can be rough, but if we can understand what is happening, it may help to make it a successful experience.

Oxytocin is the hormone responsible for moving milk from the breast ducts to the nipples and allows the bond between the mother and baby to build. At the same time, oxytocin helps the uterus to contract. It is also produced when we are sexually aroused and fall in love, hence its name "the love hormone." With all this in mind, it's no wonder breastfeeding is so crucial for both mother and baby.

I also co-slept for the first year, which is certainly a controversial topic in this country, but it felt so natural for me. My baby, like all babies, wanted more than anything to be always near me, and sleeping together was one of the best ways to achieve this. If you think about it, mammals are the same. They sleep right next to their mother. Co-sleeping allowed both of us, and my husband, to sleep well, since we weren't waking up to walk across the house every few hours to feed the baby. I personally think it is one of the most underrated ways to achieve connection with our baby and help with postpartum recovery, both mentally and physically.

When we sleep with our baby, we sleep more soundly, and the baby is more content because he is close to his mother. If we can sleep better, we feel better during the day, and are less likely to suffer from postpartum depression. Co-sleeping is widely practiced in many other parts of the world.[5] In Japan, for example, co-sleeping is the norm,[6] and the country has one of the lowest rates of infant mortality.[7] On the other hand, in the US, we have a fairly high rate of infant mortality,[8] yet we typically do not co-sleep and are strongly discouraged from doing so by our medical providers.

Fast-forward years later, and I'll never forget leaving to go home from the hospital with my third child. The pediatrician, whom I had never met and was just completing her rounds for the day, came by to meet with me and my son before we could be discharged. She asked me if I had a crib or what sleeping arrangements I was planning for the baby. I mentioned that I co-sleep and had done so with my last two babies as well. Her look of horror and implication that I was intentionally harming my baby was so offensive that to this day when I think about it, I am still frustrated and disappointed by her response. Our medical system is doing a disservice to our mothers by treating them this way. Now obviously there are some mothers who shouldn't co-sleep due to unsafe conditions, and the specifics of the bedroom and who else is sleeping in the bed should be evaluated. The postpartum phase is a great time to have a nurse come into the home, as happens in many European countries, to evaluate sleeping arrangements and do regular checks on mom and baby.[9]

How to Make a Healthy Baby before Conception and after Birth

The first decade of life is so important. It starts from before we were ever conceived. If your mother was healthy before she became pregnant—not on any medications, ate a healthy diet, took fish oil and prenatal vitamins—then you were likely set up for a healthy body. If you were delivered vaginally, breastfed, not separated from your mother for any reason, and were a full-term baby, then you had a very good running start. I was a C-section baby, and therefore my gut microbiome was negatively affected at birth. But I was breastfed for nine months, so that definitely helped. Sometimes, not all of these things are feasible, but if we can pay attention to these factors and achieve as many as possible, then we are giving our baby a healthy beginning.

Within the first few years of life, there are many factors that can impact a child's overall health. For instance, many babies are given Tylenol for fevers or antibiotics for recurrent ear infections. And vaccinations can affect their immune system as well. Combined, these things change the gut microbiome, which influences hormones and our susceptibility to depression and anxiety later in life, as our serotonin levels are made in our gut. Changes in the gut microbiome also affect our immune system, as about 70 percent of the cells found in the immune system originate in the gut. The gut microbiome begins to develop in childhood, and it reaches the diversity that is found in an adult by around the age of five.[10]

Chronic stress also causes disruption in the development of the child. The prolonged release of cortisol (the stress hormone) leads to downregulation of thyroid hormone, growth hormone, and insulin-like growth factor (IGF-1), which in turn can affect growth.[11]

Exposure to antibiotics: I realize there are times when antibiotics are needed, which is the case throughout life, but in general, they are prescribed far more than necessary. Most respiratory viruses and ear infections will resolve on their own and do not need antibiotics. If you can avoid giving your child antibiotics, it is best for their growth and development. I personally reserve antibiotics for severe bacterial infections, if my children ever have one. Thus, in cases of mild infection I usually do supportive care such as cold baths if they have a fever, along with rest, healthy foods, and vitamins to support their immune system. It's worked for our family thus far.

Food: Avoid dairy. Most cow's milk sold in grocery stores has antibiotics and toxins that disrupt the gut microbiome. This disruption leads to inflammation and gut dysbiosis,[12] which can trigger asthma, eczema, type 1 diabetes, and obesity.[13] Gluten can also be highly inflammatory. If your child has gut issues or autoimmune diseases, cut out dairy and gluten and load up on vegetables and fruit. Sugar is also in packaged foods and is overconsumed. It is very addictive for children. This, along with food dyes and processed foods, can cause behavior disruption, and ADHD and hyperactivity. This then leads children to being placed on medication due to their inability to focus. Change a child's diet and see how their behavior changes.

Here is a great list of foods my nutritionist recommends:

Antioxidants: Eat foods like berries, citrus fruit, cherries, and pomegranates. I love to make my kids smoothies to get them all in.

Foods high in omega-3 fatty acids: Salmon, nuts, avocado, and eggs.

Sufficient amount of protein: As a building block of muscles and cells, sufficient protein is needed by kids for proper growth. Organic chicken, fish, beef, eggs, lentils, and beans are all good sources.

Exercise: Exercise is key for psychological, emotional, and physical health. Several studies have found that community sports improve a child's depressive symptoms and social interactions.[14] I recommend children get outside every day. I also recommend team sports as a great way to get exercise outside of school and create a social network. It is an opportunity for children to build their self-esteem, learn the importance of teamwork, and lower stress, all while getting regular physical activity.

Regular exercise plays a crucial role in improving a child's hormonal balance. Physical activity stimulates the production of endorphins, which are hormones that help reduce stress and promote a sense of well-being. Exercise also supports the regulation of insulin levels and the production of growth hormones, which are essential for healthy development and metabolic function in children. By engaging in physical activities such as running, swimming, and playing sports, children can maintain a balanced hormonal profile, contributing to their overall physical and mental health.

Sleep: Sleep is so important for children, and parents should do all they can to prioritize it. Children should avoid caffeine, and screens should be limited, especially in the evening. This is a highly researched topic that has shown the negative impact screen time has on sleep. Dr. Jean Twenge, a professor of psychology at San Diego State University, is known for her research on the impact of digital media on mental health and well-being. Her studies have extensively examined how screen time affects sleep and other aspects of psychological health, particularly among children and adolescents. One study by Twenge looked at over forty-seven thousand children ages zero to seventeen years old and found that children who spent multiple hours on electronic devices had shorter sleep durations.[15] A review of sixty-seven published studies revealed that 90 percent of the studies found a negative correlation between screen time and sleep quality (primarily shortened duration and delayed onset).[16]

In addition to these findings, sleep is crucial for maintaining a child's hormonal balance. During deep sleep, the body releases growth hormone, which is essential for development and physical growth in children. Adequate sleep helps regulate cortisol levels (the stress hormone). Proper cortisol levels ensure that children can handle stress better and maintain emotional balance. Sleep also plays a role in the regulation of insulin and other metabolic hormones, contributing to a healthy metabolism and reducing the risk of developing conditions like obesity and diabetes. Ensuring that children get enough restful sleep is therefore fundamental not just for their immediate well-being but also for their long-term health and hormonal balance.

Toxins/chemical exposure: A few years ago, I had a patient whose son was newly diagnosed with autism. She couldn't understand why this perfectly healthy and smart boy had suddenly displayed signs of regression and learning disabilities. She started to analyze her child's environment and realized that he was in a school that backed up to a golf course where herbicides were used on a regular basis. She took him out of school, and within a few weeks, his signs of regression began to fade. His personality returned and he no longer had learning difficulties.

Chemical exposure can disrupt a child's hormonal balance in several ways. Endocrine-disrupting chemicals (EDCs) like glyphosate can interfere with the endocrine system. These chemicals mimic or block hormones and disrupt the body's normal functions. For example, glyphosate has been shown to affect the balance of sex hormones such as estrogen and testosterone,[17] potentially leading to developmental and reproductive issues.

Exposure to certain household cleaners that contain EDCs, such as phthalates and bisphenol A (BPA), can also wreak havoc on hormones. These substances can lead to altered levels of hormones that regulate growth, metabolism, and mood. In children, this can manifest as developmental delays, behavioral issues, and other health problems. Research has linked early exposure to these chemicals with a range of adverse effects, including obesity, diabetes, and thyroid dysfunction.[18]

Parents should be vigilant about the potential sources of chemical exposure in their children's environments. Using nontoxic cleaning products and being mindful of pesticide use can help minimize these risks and support better hormonal health for children. Check the products that your children are exposed to both in and around your house. Whenever possible, make sure they are nontoxic. There's a vast array of nontoxic cleaners on the market now, so it doesn't require much research to find some great options.*

Social Support and Parenting Classes:

When my three children were born, I took parenting classes at our local church and found them very helpful. They were taught by a seasoned mother of six, and she was so wonderful in guiding me through the ups and downs of the early stages of babyhood. It was also reassuring to listen to fellow mothers who were in the same season of life and hear their suggestions and perspectives. I would highly recommend something like this, especially for first-time mothers.

In addition to the social support found in parenting classes, here are a few key takeaways you can gain from them, and the wonderful impact they can have on your child, including his or her hormonal balance:

---

* You can learn more about safe cleaning products on the Environmental Working Group's website: https://www.ewg.org/cleaners/.

1. *Stress Reduction:*

   Parenting classes often educate parents on effective strategies for managing stress and fostering a calm home environment. Lower stress levels in the mother can lead to lower stress levels in children, especially babies, which is crucial for maintaining balanced cortisol levels. Babies really pick up on the mother's stress. Chronic stress and elevated cortisol can disrupt their various hormonal functions, including growth and metabolism.

2. *Consistent Routines:*

   You'll likely learn the importance of consistent routines, such as regular sleep schedules and balanced nutrition. As mentioned, proper sleep and nutrition are fundamental for hormonal regulation. Consistent sleep routines help maintain melatonin and growth-hormone levels, which are essential for a child's development.

3. *Positive Emotional Environment:*

   These classes teach parents how to provide emotional support and recognize the emotional needs of their children. A stable emotional environment can promote the production of oxytocin, which plays a role in bonding and stress reduction. Oxytocin can positively influence emotional regulation and stress resilience in children.

4. *Healthy Lifestyle Habits:*
   You'll learn about physical activities and outdoor play, which are vital for a child's physical health and hormonal balance. As covered earlier in the chapter, exercise promotes the release of endorphins, improving mood and reducing stress, and supports the regulation of growth hormones and other metabolic hormones.

5. *Awareness of Environmental Toxins:*
   Some parenting classes teach you how to be aware of potential environmental toxins (like pesticides and household cleaners). As I shared, lower exposure to these toxins supports a healthier hormonal balance and reduces the risk of developmental and reproductive issues.

Dr. Taylor's Checklist

- Exercise is key for children. Be active, get outside, be in nature. Explore.

- Whenever possible, breastfeed for at least one year. Don't be discouraged if it is painful at first. Seek help from your OB/Gyn or midwife.

- Whenever possible, try to have a vaginal delivery. Finding a holistic OB/Gyn or midwife can help to create a natural and engaging experience for both you and your baby.

- Co-sleeping. Although controversial in the US, I believe co-sleeping is a perfectly healthy option for most mothers and babies.

  Note: There are guidelines that you should follow, such as co-sleeping on a firm mattress, making sure your baby's head isn't covered, and ensuring your baby isn't sleeping in a way where they can roll off the bed. I always slept with my baby in the middle, between my husband and me, and this worked well for us.

- Take prenatal vitamins and omega-3 fatty acids during pregnancy and avoid medications as much as possible. I used Metagenics for my prenatal vitamins and loved their easy one-a-day pack that had everything I needed.

- Avoid a stressful environment as much as possible, both during pregnancy and in the early years of childhood, because cortisol production in your child hinders healthy growth and development. Be intentional about taking time for you and your child to relax daily.

- Avoid chemicals and toxins in household products.

- Limit dairy and gluten.

- Limit artificial sweeteners, food dyes, processed foods, and sugary foods and drinks.

- Feed your child's gut with probiotics, fiber, fruits and vegetables, and water.

- Prioritize sleep and create healthy sleep routines.

- Parent education classes can help you to connect with your baby. Find one at your local church or community center.

Chapter 3

YOUR TEENS

Your body starts to change in your teen years. This is when puberty begins, and the menstrual cycle can wreak havoc on a young woman's life. Heavy periods, migraines, mood swings like anxiety and depression, suicidal thoughts, and acne are all signs of hormone mayhem.

Your Menstrual Cycle

I think it's important to understand the phases of your cycle, so let's start with the basics:

Follicular Phase: The follicular phase begins on day 1 of your period (the day you start bleeding) and ends when you ovulate. It commonly lasts about fourteen days but often varies and can be shorter or longer. It starts when the hypothalamus sends a signal to your pituitary gland to release follicle-stimulating hormone (FSH, one of the markers I test for in my menopausal patients since levels rise as we enter menopause). This stimulates your ovaries to produce around five to twenty small sacs called *follicles*. Each follicle contains an immature egg. Only the healthiest egg will eventually mature. The rest of the follicles will be reabsorbed into your body. The maturing follicle sets off an estrogen surge that thickens the lining of your uterus. This creates a nutrient-rich environment for an embryo to grow.

Ovulation Phase: Rising estrogen levels during the follicular phase trigger your pituitary gland to release luteinizing hormone (LH). This, in turn, starts the process of ovulation, which is when your ovary releases a mature egg. The egg travels down the fallopian tube toward the uterus to be fertilized by sperm. Ovulation occurs right in the middle of your menstrual cycle, around day 14 if you have a twenty-eight-day cycle. It lasts about twenty-four hours. After a day, the egg will die or dissolve if it isn't fertilized.

Luteal phase: After the follicle releases its egg, it changes into the corpus luteum, which releases progesterone and some estrogen. The rise in progesterone keeps your uterine lining thick and ready for a fertilized egg to implant. If you do get pregnant, your body will produce human chorionic gonadotropin (hCG). This is the hormone that pregnancy tests are designed to detect. The hCG helps maintain the corpus luteum and keeps the uterine lining thick. However, if you don't get pregnant, the corpus luteum will shrink and be resorbed. This leads to a drop in both estrogen and progesterone, which causes the onset of your period, or the menstrual cycle. The key here is this: if the progesterone falls too low, or you were already deficient, your estrogen will become dominant and symptoms of premenstrual syndrome (PMS) may occur (see the next section for more on this). Like the follicular phase, the duration of the luteal phase can vary, lasting from eleven to seventeen days.

Common Menstrual Cycle Maps*

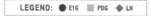

Example 1

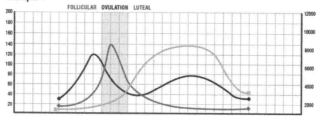

Ovulatory Menstrual Cycle

This is an average menstrual cycle. The cycle is marked by a clear LH peak with a corresponding rise in estrogen showing a strong ovulation. There is a strong rise in progesterone and a secondary rise in estrogen peaking halfway between ovulation and the first day of the next period. A sudden drop of estrogen **and progesterone occurs just prior to the start of the next period.**

Example 2

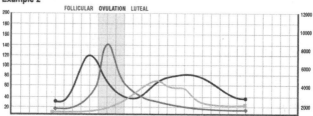

Luteal Phase Defect Cycle

This cycle shows a clear LH peak with an associated luteal phase rise in estrogen. However, progesterone rises to a lower level than normal, resulting in a lower Pg/E2 ratio. This imbalance of progesterone and estrogen in the luteal phase can lead to symptoms of estrogen dominance, PMS symptons, earlier menses, or spotting before menses.

---

* Special thanks to ZRT Laboratories for giving me permission to share these informative graphs with you.

The top graph shows an average ovulatory menstrual cycle. In the bottom graph, you can see that in the luteal phase, progesterone drops too low and estrogen dominance occurs, which can lead to mood swings, headaches, depression, and anxiety.

Hormone Imbalance and PMS

If you've ever experienced symptoms of PMS, you know how miserable they can be. It's important to recognize what the symptoms are and how to address them. Currently in our medical society, teenage girls who have PMS are usually prescribed birth control. If they have hormonal acne, they are prescribed birth control and perhaps an antibiotic or Accutane, if the acne persists. If they have depression, they might be started on an antidepressant like Zoloft. If they are suicidal, they are sent straight to a psychiatrist and, in the most severe cases, to a psychiatric ward at a hospital.

When I first started practicing medicine, I had a middle-aged woman who came to see me for several years. She was a professor and we would often talk about work or family. I'll never forget one time when she came in for a routine appointment, she told me that her daughter had been admitted to a psychiatric ward. When I asked for more details about the hospital admission, she told me that her daughter had actually been admitted several times. I couldn't believe it. When I dug a little further and asked about her period (my natural thought process when it comes to mood disorders in women), it turned out that every time her daughter was admitted, her period would start the next day. To me, the answer was obvious. She had dramatic swings in her hormones related to her cycle, and this major fluctuation was not being addressed. Psych meds weren't really helping because the root cause of her severe depression wasn't being treated.

During a similar encounter with a new patient, we were discussing family, and when my patient was telling me about her daughter, she said that she had been through a lot regarding her daughter's mental health. The mother (my patient) went on to say that her daughter had been in and out of hospitals and seen psychiatrists many times. When I asked about her cycles, similar to my other patient's daughter, as soon as she would be admitted to the hospital, the next day she would start her period.

It is startling to know the disconnect that exists between mental health in these young women and hormonal fluctuations. Psychiatrists need to understand that hormones are often at play and need to be evaluated and treated.

My takeaway for you is this: when your daughter comes to you complaining of feeling sad, or not having enough energy to get through the day, or is uninterested in hobbies or friends; when she's feeling anxious, nervous, scared, timid; or if she's dealing with acne or weight gain, headaches/migraines, cramps, or heavy periods, please think first about her hormones. These are all hormone-related symptoms. They are not just the normal experiences of modern teen life. We are not required to "grin and bear" these things. Your daughter can and should be evaluated by a physician who seriously understands hormones and can evaluate and treat her imbalance. She should not and does not have to live a miserable life. She does not need Motrin every month, or an antidepressant, or acne medication.

Furthermore, she likely does not need oral contraceptive pills (OCPs). In fact, a nationwide prospective cohort study of more than one million women living in Denmark showed an increased risk for first use of an antidepressant and first diagnosis of depression in patients using hormonal contraception, with the highest rates among adolescents.[19] I have had many patients who suffered depression as a result of birth control pills, which cause a dramatic decrease in their natural progesterone and have a severe impact on mood. If you've ever been prescribed OCPs, were you told it decreased progesterone and that depression is a possible side effect?

The topic of preventing an unwanted birth is a conversation that comes up often in my practice, and when my patients are looking for a good birth control method, I frequently recommend the copper IUD, which is nonhormonal. In addition to being aware of your cycle and when you ovulate, a nonhormonal IUD is a better option than OCPs for most patients.

Common PMS Symptoms to Watch For

Heavy bleeding, another very common symptom of PMS in teens (and other ages), is caused by estrogen dominance. How do you define heavy bleeding? I assess this by asking my patient one question: How often do you change your pad or tampon? If the answer is every two hours or less, that is considered heavy bleeding. I once had a patient tell me she changed her tampon every thirty minutes. This had been going on for years and she just figured it was normal. That is an incredible loss of blood. This kind of heavy bleeding is a significant sign of hormone imbalance and is a clear indication that hormones need to be evaluated and addressed.

Migraines are often a symptom of PMS as well. It's amazing how many women suffer from migraines. Looking back on my high school years, I had a classmate who would get migraines. I'll never forget seeing her head on the desk in math class. As I think about it now, I realize that she very likely had migraines related to her periods.

Migraines can be very debilitating, and the

main route for treatment for teenagers or women of any age is to start on prescription medication. But what if your migraines are related to your periods? What if they are a sign that your hormones are off? What if fixing your hormones fixed your migraines? It's very possible it will.

In my medical opinion, hormones should be the very first thing that is evaluated in a menstruating woman of any age. For these patients, I start with a blood test and an at-home saliva or urine test kit. Depending on when they have migraines, I might test with a thirty-day menstrual map that looks at their estrogen and progesterone fluctuations throughout the month. It is a great tool for analyzing PMS related to a shift in estrogen and progesterone and can help determine when a hormone imbalance should be addressed. A menstrual map is especially good for women who get migraines at different times during their cycle, depending on how their estrogen rises and falls. They may have migraines at ovulation when there is an estrogen surge, or during the last half of their cycle when their progesterone falls. The menstrual map gives me information about the fluctuation in hormones throughout the month. If an estrogen rise occurs, DIM (diindolylmethane) is a great supplement that I use to help regulate estrogen.[20] If progesterone is low, chasteberry extract can help increase progesterone. Diet is also key, and I usually recommend an anti-inflammatory diet—avoiding sugar, gluten, dairy, and alcohol.

Sometimes an allergy test can be helpful to determine if there is a food or environmental exposure (think mycotoxins from mold) that could be contributing to migraines. The point is, there may be a few things that need to be addressed. It's important to know that meds are *not* the first line of defense. All other avenues should be considered and evaluated prior to prescribing medication.

To summarize, having a period is not a diagnosis. It is not something for which medication should be required. PMS is not, nor should be, the norm. The most likely culprit of your daughter's PMS symptoms is that her progesterone is too low for her—not determined by a reference range on a blood test but rather by what she needs specifically for her physiological makeup. She may need an oral form of progesterone or she may need a cream application; she may need a low dose or a higher dose; and she may need it for a few days or a couple of weeks out of the month. It just really depends on what works best for her. But the answer should be very clear: she likely has a hormone imbalance.

Functional Medicine and PMS

So what should you expect from your functional medicine practitioner when it comes to PMS? Here is what I address when evaluating the root cause of PMS:

1. **Hormone levels:** Estrogen and progesterone levels during the luteal phase is key. This will show me if estrogen is too high or progesterone is too low. Depending on when symptoms occur, I may need to look at a full thirty-day map. I also look at cortisol levels, which can increase from chronic stress and affect the hormone balance.

2. **Diet:** I ask patients for detailed food journals—because what you eat plays a huge role in your hormones. I know that can be challenging with teenagers, but the earlier they learn how food affects their body, the better.

3. **Gut:** How would your teen describe her digestive system? The questions I ask my patients are:

   a. What are your bowel movements like?

   b. Are you constipated?

   c. Are you bloated?

   d. Do you have symptoms of irritable bowel? (i.e. bloating, diarrhea or loose stools, frequent bowel movements, stress-induced bowel movements, constipation, cramping, etc.)

   These are all key factors to address what is going on with a patient's gut microbiome and digestion. No matter your age, your gut is a window into your overall health and risk for chronic diseases such as cancer and dementia.

4. **Lifestyle:** What is your teen's lifestyle like? Does she get enough sleep? Does she take time for herself, without excess input from screens, headphones, and so on?

5. **Stress:** What is her current stress level and how is she dealing with it? Does she have a healthy outlet to decrease her stress?

6. **Allergies:** Does she have allergies? Food? Seasonal?

7. **Environment:** Could your teen be ingesting or exposed to something every day that you aren't even aware of that is causing symptoms? Has she ever been exposed to mold? Has your family ever lived in a home that flooded? Could mold be lurking in her school's air ducts?

This type of analysis takes time that most doctors don't have in abundance. However, it is this full-picture analysis of a patient that will provide the keys needed to appropriately analyze specific symptoms. Whereas many physicians will just zero in on the symptom and find ways to manage it (a Band-Aid approach), a functional medicine doctor wants to get to the root cause of the symptom and address it directly. This leads to long-lasting relief. This should be the standard of care in medicine.

Natural Solutions for PMS Symptoms

Okay, let's talk solutions. Often the first strategy for relieving PMS symptoms is to balance estrogen and progesterone, but there are many other things that can be done to help. I prefer to start with supplements to balance hormones, especially for my younger patients.

- **Chaste Tree Extract:** I love the herb Vitex (my go-to brand is Gaia Herbs), and I prescribe it often. This supplement helps raise progesterone levels, and I often recommend it for patients who have mild symptoms related to PMS. I love it when this works because it's cheap and easy.

- **Vitamin B6:** This also helps with PMS symptom relief. I recommend my patients take it throughout the month for a couple cycles to see if it makes a difference.

- **Magnesium glycinate, B-complex vitamins, D3+K2, and calcium:** These supplements can all have a measurable positive impact on PMS symptoms.

- **Exercise:** Moving the body is critical as well, and I always tell my patients to prioritize frequency over intensity. Because exercise is very personal and unique to each of us, it's important to create an exercise routine that is enjoyable and doable for you. Your teen might detest the idea of running, but she loves riding a bike or in-line skating. Yoga can also be really great for building strength and focusing the mind—and it's a great mother-daughter activity. It's worth investing the time to try different kinds of exercise until your teen finds the magic form of movement that she enjoys and that she can easily work into her schedule throughout the week.

- **Acupuncture:** This is another natural option to try, and though there is only limited data in published studies regarding its efficacy in relieving PMS symptoms, I have enough anecdotal evidence to feel confident recommending it. Make sure your acupuncturist is licensed in your state, and always ask for a phone or in-person consultation first to get an idea of the type of acupuncture he or she practices, and to make sure your teen feels a good connection with the practitioner. The more comfortable your teen feels with the acupuncturist and with the setting, the more effective the sessions will be. And be sure to clearly communicate your goals. If a reduction in PMS symptoms is your primary reason for the visit, explain that so the practitioner can focus their energy on it.

- **Diet:** What your teen eats is an incredibly important factor when it comes to regulating hormones. I always go through a complete diet survey to understand what patients are consuming on a regular basis. I especially discourage patients from eating foods that increase hormone disruption, such as dairy, sugar, gluten/wheat, and alcohol. These can have a major impact on hormones.

Insulin Resistance

This is more related to my older patients, but I want to put something else on your radar—insulin resistance. That's when cells in your muscles, fat, and liver cannot easily take up glucose from your blood. Insulin resistance is more common than you think and is often overlooked. It can cause your pancreas to increase its insulin production, which, in turn, can lead to prediabetes. I find glucose monitors to be very helpful in identifying the presence of insulin resistance or prediabetes. These are devices that are worn on the arm to evaluate glucose levels throughout the day and send you alerts on your smartphone. Glucose spikes depend on what we eat, therefore continuous glucose monitors are incredibly helpful in evaluating which foods trigger a glucose spike.

I know it's tough when talking about diet with teenagers, but I think it is extremely important for them to understand that a lot of their symptoms, whether mood, skin issues, or weight, can be addressed through diet. I know firsthand the benefits of a plant-based diet—meaning, in general, the more plants you can eat, the better. We get so many amazing nutrients from our fruits and vegetables, not to mention the fiber that comes with it, which is so important for our gut health. When possible, select locally sourced, organic produce to avoid ingesting unwanted hormones or toxic pesticides.

Water intake is critical as well. Generally, people do not drink enough water daily, which is detrimental to overall health. The target is half of your body weight in ounces. For example, if you weigh 150 pounds, you will need to consume 75 ounces of water daily. If that seems unachievable, then drinking at least 64 ounces is a good goal. Think about finding a cute stainless steel or glass (avoid plastic) water bottle that your teen loves and will keep with her throughout the day.

The Menstrual Cycle as Your Fifth Vital Sign

Have you ever heard of this concept before? When you go to the doctor for a regular checkup, they typically check your vital signs—heart rate, blood pressure, body temperature, and respiratory rate. Your cycle should be asked about and monitored in some detail. How regular your cycle is, how heavy it is, how frequently or infrequently it comes every month are all indications of your overall health. This is true for all menstruating women.

Your cycle can also tell you so much about your health and your specific disease risk factors. If your cycle is irregular, this can lead to an increased risk of diseases down the road. A study published in the *British Medical Journal* in 2020 called "The Nurses' Health Study II" looked at nearly eighty thousand premenopausal women with no history of cardiovascular disease, cancer, or diabetes, and found that women with irregular cycles had an increased risk of mortality compared to their counterparts who reported regular cycles. The study analyzed women for twenty-four years and asked them to report the usual length and regularity of their cycle at ages fourteen to seventeen years old, eighteen to twenty-two years old, and twenty-nine to forty-six years old. The leading causes of those premature deaths (before the age of seventy) were cancer and cardiovascular disease.[21]

In addition, according to an Australian database analysis, women with irregular menses were 20 percent more likely to develop cardiovascular disease and 17 percent more likely to develop type 2 diabetes over twenty years when compared with women with regular menstrual cycles.[22]

And a fifty-year prospective study of 15,528 mothers in the Child Health and Development Studies cohort recruited from the Kaiser Foundation Health Plan looked at the correlation between irregular menstrual cycles and ovarian cancer. The prevailing hypothesis had been that less frequent ovulatory cycles would reduce ovarian cancer risk, so researchers expected that irregular cycles would be protective. Instead, they found that irregular cycles were a marker for higher risk of ovarian cancer.[23] All those years, doctors thought that an irregular cycle that meant less ovulation over time was somehow healthy for a woman, when in fact, the opposite was true.

I think we can agree that the menstrual cycle is your fifth vital sign, and it's important to pay attention to what it's telling you. Are your cycles regular? The average length of a cycle is twenty-eight days; however, a normal cycle can range between twenty-one and thirty-five days, and periods should last between three and seven days. If you're falling outside of that range, it's a good idea to talk to your functional medicine doctor about why that might be.

This is just another reason taking birth control pills is so detrimental: It cuts off your access to your fifth vital sign. Even though OCP packs include a placebo week, which is the week off birth control that induces a "period," that's not an actual normal period. The whole function of birth control pills is to keep you from ovulating. So you can't really know anything about your natural menstrual cycle while you're on birth control pills. And that is the main reason I do not recommend birth control pills to my patients. It is best to allow your body to have its normal cycle. Your crucial cycle information can be used to further understand your overall health.

Dr. Taylor's Checklist
for Teens and Their Parents

1. **If acne is an issue**: Making a diet change is key. Talk to your teen about eliminating fast food, sugar, dairy, bad fats, and processed foods. Addressing the gut is important as acne can be a sign of gut microbial imbalance. And of course, having their hormones analyzed will help elucidate if a hormone imbalance (i.e., testosterone overproduction) is causing a problem. There are some great supplements to help with decreasing testosterone production, like saw palmetto. If acne continues to be an issue, spironolactone is a testosterone blocker and can be a helpful medication in the short term. This works well for teens, too, in conjunction with the aforementioned diet changes.

2. **Analyze your period**: Talk to your teen daughter about these questions: What do your periods look like? Are they bright-red blood? Are they regular? Are they heavy? Do you have cramps? Do you have mood swings? Do you have headaches? These are all signs that your daughter's hormones are off. Start with addressing diet

and gut. Cut out dairy, sugar, and gluten. I also suggest the following:

- Take Vitex.

- Drink a lot of water and cut out all other drinks, especially sugary drinks.

- Take a probiotic.

- Eat fiber such as vegetables, oats, flaxseed, beans, lentils, and fruit.

- Make sure you are having a bowel movement daily so that your hormones are not backing up into your system and causing you to have excessive hormones.

- Avoid birth control if possible as this disrupts your hormonal system completely. Consider a copper IUD if looking for a consistent form of birth control.

- Take a good multivitamin.

3. **Exercise**: Is your teen exercising regularly? Encourage them to join a sports team. They should be exercising every day for about an hour. Remember, exercise is a natural mood stabilizer.

4. **Substances**: It's so important that you talk to your teen about these questions too. Are they

drinking, doing drugs, smoking? Are they taking (or abusing) prescription meds? If so, these drugs could be making their body toxic, which affects the gut, brain, hormones, and everything in between. All these things cause inflammation in all parts of the body and lead to emotional and physical destruction.

5. **Food**: I mentioned this already, but diet is so important. Is your teen eating well? Avoiding sugary foods and drinks? Eating fast food? Eating fruits and vegetables every day? Eat well and your body and brain will thank you.

6. **Sleep:** Is your teen prioritizing sleep? Sleep helps your brain to unwind, stimulates growth hormone, and is important for your mental health. Talk to your teen about getting at least eight to nine hours of sleep each night. If needed, rearrange schedules for the next month so that your teen can reach that threshold, then see how much better they feel.

7. **Stress:** Stress can be a big issue among teens with academic and social pressures. Limiting or avoiding social media can be key in preventing social stress. Teaching our teens how to manage

their time and get academic help early and often can help to mitigate pressure related to school. Parents need to keep a close eye on their children and evaluate how they are spending their time. Practicing a consistent exercise that focuses on releasing tension—such as running, swimming, and yoga—can help to reduce stress.

8. **Social connections:** How is your teen finding social outlets? Do they have good friends, a church or spiritual group? Do they have mentors they can rely on? If not, then spend some time discovering what you enjoy and look for a club that supports that. Some ideas are painting or pottery, gardening, yoga, reading, running, hiking, biking, or cooking. The possibilities are endless.

9. **Mood:** Watch your teen's mood. Her diet, gut, activity level, and sleep quality are instrumental in keeping her mood balanced. If your teen's mood is suffering, address these four areas. And remind her—never suffer in silence. Reassure her that she can come to you if she's experiencing mood swings or can't get a handle on how she's feeling.

10. **Beware of energy drinks:** They are filled with chemicals, dyes, and additives and can make things a lot worse. Talk to your teen about finding natural, healthy ways to boost her energy and never turning to chemical-laden drinks.

Chapter 4

YOUR TWENTIES

The twenties are a time of transition for most people. Whether it's finishing school or finding your first job, deciding what you want to do with your life can feel overwhelming. This can lead to immense stress, which can cause behaviors that result in damage down the road.

Stress reduction is key at any age because excessive amounts of stress can cause dysfunction no matter how old you are. But did you know that healthy stress management is also a critical factor for balancing hormones? People who routinely experience high stress are more likely to release cortisol in higher concentrations than normal, stealing resources from making estrogen and progesterone.

This effect is often referred to as the "cortisol steal."

I once had a patient who grew up in Kosovo during the war. When she came to see me in her thirties, she was experiencing significant effects of stress that were evident in her test results. All of her hormones were low, which was affecting her mood, energy, periods, and, most importantly for her, her ability to get pregnant. She was considering leaving her partner and her job. She was miserable. She came to see me to figure out if something underlying was the problem. With the necessary testing and treatment, she was finally able to feel better for the first time in decades. If you feel like stress has been a significant part of your life at one point or another, here is what to do.

The first step is to get your cortisol tested. The gold standard is a saliva test taken at four different points throughout the day. This will show whether you have spikes during the day, and likewise whether you have dips.

If your cortisol is out of balance, I recommend proper stress management. I always think it's interesting how specific test results and symptoms correlate. I will often see a patient's test results show that their cortisol is too low in the morning, a sign of adrenal fatigue (more on that later). When I ask if they wake up dragging, they almost always say yes. Likewise, if I see a spike in the evening, that almost always correlates with stress that ensues around dinnertime—just getting home from work and dealing with a spouse or roommates. Adrenal support and stress management can be extremely helpful at times during the day when cortisol spikes. I always encourage my patients to find ways to manage their stress by doing something they enjoy and that relaxes them, whether it's yoga, walking, gardening, prayer, meditation, or something else. I love the app Headspace, which is a wonderful tool to guide deep-breathing exercises. Whatever it is that works, it's important to be consistent with stress management.

What Is Adrenal Fatigue?

The importance of stress management and healing the adrenals should not be taken lightly. Let's look closely at the adrenals: they are small, triangular-shaped glands above the kidneys that are important for regulating blood pressure, immune function, and the body's response to stress. In an emergency situation—your house is on fire, for example—the adrenals produce cortisol to respond to stress. But it is meant to be produced in short spurts. When the body is in a chronic state of stress, cortisol is produced over long periods of time.

Overproduction of cortisol leads to fatigue, poor sleep, depression, anxiety, weight gain, sugar cravings, and addiction, among other things. Healing the adrenals includes addressing stress, sleep, relaxation, and adrenal support with supplements. And if you can get a handle on all of this in your twenties, you'll set yourself up for better managing life's stressors as you age.

Gut Health and Why It's So Important

I touched on the gut microbiome in earlier chapters, and that's because your gut is a huge piece of your body's hormone puzzle throughout your lifetime.

If your gut is out of balance, it really impacts your hormones, not to mention everything else. Think about this: imbalances with the gut microbiome are the root of many autoimmune diseases; in fact, this is one of the first places I look when a patient comes to me with an autoimmune diagnosis. Many autoimmune diseases, like fibromyalgia and lupus, are due to a gut imbalance.[24]

Gut imbalance also causes the recirculation of hormones, thus leading to estrogen dominance. Interestingly, that's often how women become estrogen-dominant. Women are supposed to excrete excess estrogen, but with a leaky gut, the hormones get recirculated back into their blood stream. This can lead to ovarian cysts, fibroids, and endometriosis, to name a few. For every woman with signs of hormone imbalance like PMS, their gut microbiome should be analyzed with a stool and breath test.

So what are signs that your gut is out of balance? Constipation is an important clue. Many of my patients have gone years having irregular bowel movements, sometimes not eliminating for days at a time. This is not normal. Having a regular bowel movement every day is normal and should be the goal. If you are not having a bowel movement every day, your gut is not working properly. The toxins and hormones that should be excreted from your body on a daily basis are sitting idle, and this is not healthy.

When we talk about gut health, many of my patients immediately assume they just need to start taking probiotics, but that is not necessarily the case. In fact, popping a probiotic pill every day can make matters worse for you. For example, if you have SIBO (or small-intestine bacterial overgrowth) and you take probiotics, you're just feeding the overgrowth and your symptoms can get worse. If you are taking a probiotic and your symptoms are worsening or not improving, it can be a sign that you have SIBO and you should do further testing. A full analysis of the bacterial makeup of your gut will show precisely what needs to be corrected in order to get your microbiome on track and restore your gut health.

Anti-Inflammatory Diet

An anti-inflammatory diet is a great starting place for anyone, and if you get in the habit of eating this way while you're in your twenties, you'll be putting yourself on a path of wellness for the rest of your life. Ridding your diet of inflammatory foods—including dairy, gluten, alcohol, and sugar—can make a major difference, even without making any other lifestyle changes. Getting your body to be less inflamed is a very important first step.

I often recommend patients begin by cutting out gluten. It can take a good four to six weeks to notice a difference, but the improvement—from increased energy to better sleep and improved depression or anxiety symptoms—can be huge.

Annie Mabashov is the certified Functional Diagnostic Nutrition Practitioner (FDN-P) and Integrative Health Coach (IHC) that works with me to see all my patients for their dietary and lifestyle needs. She's brilliant at helping design realistic, anti-inflammatory nutrition plans.

As a cancer survivor, Annie knows firsthand the impact that functional-based nutrition and lifestyle changes can have to help regain your health. After completing chemo in 2013 for stage IV Hodgkin's lymphoma, Annie was cancer-free, but she still struggled with a weakened immune system, chronic fatigue, and recurrent infections. Allopathic medicine provided some instant relief from some of these symptoms but did not provide long-term solutions to rebuilding health.

Annie then became fascinated with the power of nutrition, specifically anti-inflammatory diets and living a cleaner lifestyle. She also started seeing a functional medicine doctor who took the time to go through functional lab work and put her on a protocol that changed her life and gave her back the vitality she had lost through the course of her illness.

An anti-inflammatory diet involves eating nutrient-rich, whole foods that reduce inflammation in the body. It contains plenty of fiber, antioxidants, and omega-3 fatty acids. This means a diet rich in vegetables, whole fruit, complex carbohydrates, legumes, lean proteins, and fatty fish, and one that is as unprocessed as possible.

Benefits of an anti-inflammatory diet include:

1. reduction of chronic disease,
2. better blood sugar control, and
3. improved heart health.

For the purposes of this book, I asked Annie to share her anti-inflammatory food list so you could start to think about how to eat in this way. Here's her list:

1. Fatty fish: Salmon, mackerel, sardines, and trout are rich in omega-3 fatty acids.

2. Berries: Strawberries, blueberries, raspberries, and blackberries contain antioxidants like anthocyanins.

3. Leafy greens: Spinach, kale, and Swiss chard are high in vitamins and antioxidants.

4. Cruciferous vegetables: Cauliflower, broccoli, cabbage, and bok choy are packed with antioxidants, which help neutralize free radicals and reduce oxidative stress, a contributor to chronic inflammation.

5. Nuts and seeds: Almonds, walnuts, chia seeds, and flaxseeds provide healthy fats and fiber.

6. Olive oil: Extra virgin olive oil has powerful anti-inflammatory effects.

7. Turmeric: Contains curcumin, a powerful anti-inflammatory compound.

8. Ginger: Ginger is known for its anti-inflammatory and antioxidant effects.

9. Garlic: Garlic contains sulfur compounds that exhibit anti-inflammatory properties.

10. Green Tea: This tea is rich in polyphenols and antioxidants.

11. Peppers: Bell peppers and chili peppers are high in vitamin C and antioxidants.

12. Avocados: This fruit provides healthy fats and antioxidants.

If you'd like to discover some delicious recipes or learn more about Annie, visit WellwithAnnie.com. Thanks, Annie.

I encourage you to focus on the previous list of foods to include in your diet and, as you do, to start limiting or eliminating these foods:

1. **Gluten:** Gluten molecules increase intestinal permeability, allowing toxins into the blood stream and causing inflammation in the gut in particular and the body in general.

2. **Dairy:** Sixty-five percent of the world is lactose intolerant.[25] Most people do not have the enzyme to break down dairy. Dairy is highly inflammatory and difficult to digest properly and should be avoided.

3. **Sugar:** Promotes oxidative stress and inflammation by damaging cells and tissues.

4. **Refined/Artificial Foods:** Stimulate an immune response, leading to increased production of pro-inflammatory cytokines.

5. **Alcohol:** Alcohol consumption generates reactive molecules that can damage cells, proteins, and DNA, leading to oxidative stress and inflammation.

If you are unsure how to incorporate an anti-inflammatory diet into your lifestyle, it may be helpful to start by shopping for organic, plant-based, and whole foods, or find a food delivery service that offers an anti-inflammatory meal program. These services can be expensive, but if preparation or time is a concern, you might try it for just a few months for ideas on how to put meals together. In general, as I've noted, sticking to a non-processed, plant-based diet is key.

On this topic, I love the movie *Forks over Knives*.[26] I first watched it when I was a resident at Loma Linda University in my preventive medicine program. It is an incredible documentary that shows the impact of diet on our health. It shows how we can reverse and prevent the diseases that plague our society simply by changing what we eat. One of the key contributors to the movie is Dr. Caldwell Esselstyn, a cardiologist at the Cleveland Clinic. He works with complex and complicated cardiac patients who are beyond surgical repair. His incredible and revolutionary approach focuses on adopting a plant-based diet. It is fascinating and also so logical to me at the same time. We tend to overcomplicate things in our medical world, but if we bring things back to the basics of healthy living, the body adjusts accordingly. I have heard Dr. Esselstyn speak in person several times and am intrigued every time I listen to his story and the way in which he reverses disease in his patients. He and his entire family have devoted their lives to educating people to eat better and live better. If you haven't seen the film, I highly recommend it.

While we're on the topic of nutrition, I'd like to mention that for my patients who have an elevated fasting glucose or are at risk for diabetes, I often recommend they wear a continuous glucose monitor for a few weeks or even a few months. This is incredibly helpful data for determining which foods are causing glucose to be elevated. I have had patients make major strides in homing in on their diet and increasing weight loss in the process. The point is, collecting data is important when it comes to figuring out what aspects of your life are having a direct impact on your hormones.

Birth Control Pills

I have worked with so many patients who regret their decision to go onto birth control when they were in their twenties because of the long-lasting negative effects it's had on their hormones. So, if you're a twentysomething right now and you're either already taking birth control or plan to begin, I want to help you understand how this might be affecting your health.

Let's begin by looking for a moment at the history of birth control pills. I think seeing the timeline is helpful in understanding how OCPs (oral contraceptive pills) became the standard of care.

1916: On October 16, 1916, Margaret Sanger opened the first American birth control clinic in Brooklyn. But nine days after it opened, undercover female police officers posed as patients, shut down the clinic, and arrested Sanger.[27]

1921: Sanger established the American Birth Control League, a precursor to Planned Parenthood.

1923: Sanger opened the first doctor-staffed birth control clinic in the US.

1956: Gynecologist John Rock and biologist Gregory Pincus (with the backing of Sanger) conducted large-scale clinical trials in Puerto Rico, where there were no anti–birth control laws. The pill was deemed "100 percent effective," but some serious side effects were ignored; three women in the trial even died.[28]

1957: The first oral contraceptive, Enovid, was approved by the FDA for menstrual disorders. It contained 10 mg of norethynodrel and 150 µg of mestranol, *much* higher hormone doses than those in later formulations.

1960: Enovid was approved by the FDA as the first oral contraceptive pill.

1962: In less than two years, 1.2 million women were on the Pill, and by 1965 over 5 million women were using it. Even though the original Pill contained very high doses of synthetic estrogen and synthetic progesterone (progestin), causing an array of side effects, women preferred it to other methods like the diaphragm, condoms, and douches.[29] (By the way, did you know that women used Lysol and other antiseptics as douches to prevent pregnancy?[30])

1961–1969: Enovid faced scrutiny due to side effects such as blood clots, leading to Senate hearings called the Nelson Pill Hearings, led by Senator Gaylord Nelson.[31] By 1969, the dosage in birth control pills was reduced to lower health risks.

1980s: Dosage in birth control pills continued to be reduced to decrease side effects like blood clots. Modern birth control pills (BCPs) contain much lower levels of estrogen and progestin (synthetic progesterone) compared to those earlier versions.

1990s: Birth control pills became available in various formulations, including lower doses and combination pills with both estrogen and progestin.

2000s: Development of lower-dose pills continued, and new delivery methods, such as the contraceptive patch and vaginal ring, were introduced. Controversies emerged over birth control pills like Yaz and Yasmin. Studies found a higher risk of blood clots compared to older pills. Bayer faced around eleven thousand lawsuits, resulting in nearly $2 billion in settlements for claims involving blood clots, heart attacks, strokes, and gallbladder injuries.[32]

2009: The FDA issued warnings to Bayer for misleading advertisements that downplayed the risks of Yaz and Yasmin. Bayer was required to fund $20 million in corrective advertising.[33]

2010s: Extended-cycle pills were introduced. Women taking them had fewer periods per year. Legal and medical discussions about the safety and side effects of hormonal contraceptives were ongoing.

2017: Lawsuits emerged targeting extended-cycle pills, Seasonique and Seasonale, produced by Teva Pharmaceuticals. The cases alleged that the pills caused hepatic adenomas (liver tumors), some of which turned cancerous. Users reported severe health issues such as liver cancer, leading to multiple surgeries, including liver transplants. These cases highlighted the lack of sufficient warnings about the potential risks of liver damage from these contraceptives, highlighting the broader concerns over hormonal contraceptives and their potential side effects. "According to the lawsuit, Teva knew or should have known that there was a five-fold increased risk of hepatic adenomas after five to seven years of use, and a 25-fold increased risk after use longer than nine years."[34]

2023: The FDA approved Opill, the first over-the-counter daily oral contraceptive. Opill contains 0.075 mg of norgestrel, a progestin-only formulation with no estrogen. And you don't need a prescription to purchase it.[35] According to the FDA, side effects include "irregular vaginal bleeding, nausea, breast tenderness, and headaches."[36] Though they don't list mood disorders in the side effects, what I know from studying hormones for all these years is that synthetic progesterone (progestin) can cause mood disorders, including anxiety and depression.

Despite its checkered history, I can tell you firsthand that most doctors learn in medical school that "the Pill" is the number one choice in terms of family planning. It's usually a very short discussion between doctors and patients. And when would patients even have at-length discussions with their doctors about this topic? There's simply no time in today's quick and to-the-point appointments. Therefore, the Pill has been widely prescribed, and generations of women have been taking synthetic hormonal contraception. To this day, millions of women feel they have no other option for family planning.

The irony is that many women are deathly afraid of hormone replacement therapy for menopause, yet somehow synthetic birth control pills are okay in their minds. And the reason so many women are afraid of hormone replacement therapy for menopause is because studies showed that estrogen plus progestin increased risk of strokes, heart attacks, and breast cancer.[37] Although hormone replacement for menopause differs from the hormones in birth control pills, wouldn't you logically expect there to be very real and potentially dangerous side effects from those too? Why would birth control pills be exempt from deleterious side effects? It simply does not make sense.

If you take nothing else away from this chapter, I hope it's that the Pill is not without the potential for serious side effects, not only while you're taking them but later as well. The truth is, not enough studies have been conducted to really tell the whole story about how taking synthetic hormones to block ovulation month after month for years on end can impact future fertility. But just because there aren't enough studies to tell us one way or another *doesn't make the Pill safe*.

I never prescribe birth control pills to my patients. Instead, I have conversations with my patients about their family planning, and we come up with solutions that make sense for their situation as well as their health history. I do often recommend the copper IUD because it's nonhormonal. But there is no one-size-fits-all answer for this, and that's why it's imperative that you form a relationship with your functional medicine practitioner and have these real-life conversations. It's the only way to get to a solution that's the right fit for your body, your health, and your future.

Dr. Taylor's Checklist
for Your Twenties:

Stress: Check your stress levels. Be honest with yourself about this. Are you chronically stressed out? Are you making good life decisions? Take a step back if you need to in order to decide what is best for you. Don't get caught up with what everyone else is doing. Seek counsel from your mentors in life. Don't look to drugs, alcohol, or food to numb your stress.

Gut: If you are having gut symptoms as discussed in this chapter, get your gut checked for small intestinal bacterial overgrowth (SIBO) and leaky gut and follow an anti-inflammatory diet.

Birth control: If birth control is on your mind, it's imperative to build a relationship with a functional medicine practitioner that you trust, and then to have conversations about the best solution for you so that your future fertility doesn't suffer.

Chapter 5

YOUR THIRTIES:
THE INFERTILITY JOURNEY,
PREGNANCY,
AND POSTPARTUM

By now, many of my patients are married and planning for children. Therefore, I'm devoting this chapter to a conversation on fertility, infertility, pregnancy, and postpartum.

Hormones That
Affect Fertility

The first infertility patient I saw in my office was the sister of an old friend of mine from junior high. I had been in practice for a little over a year. She came in with her mom after hearing that I work with women who suffer from hormone imbalance and infertility. She had been married for a few years and had already suffered two miscarriages. She and her husband desperately wanted a child. Her doctors were unable to figure out what was wrong. "We really hope you can help us," she said. "We are desperate and just want to figure out why I keep miscarrying. It's not that I can't get pregnant. I just can't stay pregnant. I'm afraid that time is running out and I just don't know why we can't have a baby." She was perfectly healthy and had no underlying conditions.

Knowing how much hormones affect pregnancy and how low progesterone can cause repeated miscarriages, her story sounded exactly like a typical low-progesterone case, so I sent her for hormone testing and planned to see her back in my office a few weeks later. When I reviewed her labs, sure enough, her progesterone was low. I immediately started her on a vaginal suppository of progesterone, and within a couple of months, she was pregnant. I was ecstatic for her, her husband, her mom—her whole family. Now the goal was to maintain the pregnancy.

With continued progesterone and repeated testing to ensure her progesterone was at an optimum level during her first trimester, she was able to sustain her pregnancy. I'll never forget visiting her in the hospital after delivery and seeing her baby boy for the first time. I was so incredibly happy for her. She has since written a book about motherhood entitled *From My Life to Mom Life*. If you read it, you will see her medical journey with my practice in the first few chapters. I am so humbled to have been part of her story. Since then, I have seen countless infertility patients in my office, and she is one of many success stories.

Low progesterone isn't the only cause of miscarriage, but it is far more common than you might realize. Remember, if you have PMS, migraines, heavy periods, depression, or anxiety before your period, you have low progesterone until proven otherwise and could be at risk for having miscarriages. If you are interested in having a baby, get your progesterone checked by a functional medicine doctor before you get pregnant, and make sure your hormones are balanced.

Another hormone that can impact fertility is the thyroid hormone. Thyroid-stimulating hormone (TSH) is a hormone made in the brain that analyzes how much thyroid hormone is circulating. If it senses low levels, it will stimulate the thyroid gland to secrete thyroid hormone. I once had a patient tell me that according to her other medical provider, if her TSH was above 1.5 *mU/L*, she would not be able to get pregnant. Sure enough, that played out for her. A normal TSH range on a standard blood lab is 0.40–4.5 *mU/L*, so she would have been considered in the normal range if her test result was within these parameters but above 1.5 *mU/L*. For her, having a more optimal TSH was critical for her fertility.

If you are at all concerned about fertility or pregnancy, seek out a functional medicine physician who can look at your thyroid levels with a different lens and optimize you if needed. This analysis can help avoid a lot of heartache and potentially tens of thousands of dollars of infertility treatments.

Infertility in America

According to the CDC, "In the United States, 1 in 5 (19%) of married women aged 15 to 49 with no prior births are unable to get pregnant after one year of trying. About one in four (26%) of women in this group have difficulty getting pregnant or carrying a pregnancy to term."[38] Nowadays, many women suffering with infertility turn to IVF for assistance. According to the American Society for Reproductive Medicine, there were 91,771 babies born from IVF in 2022.[39] Now, consider that the cost of just one round of IVF treatment typically ranges between "$15,000 to $30,000, depending on the center and the patient's individual medication needs,"[40] and a woman under the age of thirty-five has only a 37.9 percent chance of having a full-term, normal birth weight baby after a single egg transfer IVF cycle.[41] When you do the math, hopeful mothers are spending millions upon millions of dollars in assisted reproductive technology every year. And most of the time, their efforts are, sadly, unsuccessful.

It may come as a surprise to you, but I think the vast majority of infertility struggles are a direct result of women using birth control pills during the years prior to their attempts to conceive. Think about it. Your body is designed to have your hormones work the way they naturally do. You are supposed to have a period every month. And as I've already noted, it does not count when you have a period on birth control pills. That is a "fake" period (which happens when women take the placebo pills in their pill pack, thus inducing a period). When do we ever suppress hormones in a man? When do we ever suppress their testosterone with a pill? It's crazy to think that we do this in women all the time.

Furthermore, your provider will probably never tell you that long-term birth control use may likely have a negative impact on your ability to conceive after you go off the Pill. You'd think there would be multiple studies that support this, given that oral contraception has been around since 1960. However, in 2013, when a group of Danish and American researchers, including an epidemiologist from Boston University, decided to look at long-term effects of pill use, they realized "little is known about long-term OCPs [oral contraceptive pills] and TTP [time to pregnancy]."[42]

In their NIH-funded study of 3,700 Danish women, researchers found a slight reduction in fecundability for women who used certain newer-generation oral contraceptives than for older OCPs, and for women who had first used OCPs at an early age. The research team said both of those findings warranted further study. The study's discussion section states, "The association between young age at first OCP use and reduced fecundability is notable but may partially reflect early age at first use among women with cycle irregularities. We believe this issue merits further investigation, as does our finding of slightly reduced fecundability for users of third and fourth generation OCPs."[43] Even with that said, you'll find on Boston University's School of Public Health news website in big, bold letters these words: "Long-term Oral Contraceptive Use Doesn't Hurt Fertility, Study Finds."[44]

Another study found that long-term use (greater than five years) of birth control pills decreased the endometrial lining and could lead to difficulties with pregnancies. "These findings suggest a previously unidentified adverse effect of long-term combined

OCP use in women who are anticipating future fertility."[45] I think it's important to be aware of how birth control pills can affect the body. And just because millions of women have taken oral contraceptives over the last sixty years doesn't mean they are good for you, or without detrimental effects.

So there are two factors to look at. The first (and this goes beyond just birth control pills): Why does the general population so deeply trust that what pharmaceutical companies tell them is unbiased? We look for biases in other things like gender discrimination and racial, religious, or political biases. Why, then, is the American culture around healthcare so no-questions-asked when something is prescribed?

The second factor: Birth control itself has gone largely unchanged since its creation. Dating back to ancient times, blends of herbs were concocted and ingested by women in order to prevent or end pregnancy. Fast forward to the 1950s when the first studies were conducted on women using synthetic birth control pills. The Pill saw one major improvement in the 1980s when the original high-dose pill was replaced with a much lower dose version after 6.5 million women had already been on it.[46] The majority of contraceptive advancements have taken place only in the last twenty years. Women have been trying to control when, where, and how they want to get pregnant since the beginning of time But, on a continuum of birth control advancement, we are at the very beginning of beginnings. And yet, 64.9 percent of the 72.2 million women ages fifteen to forty-nine in the US are on the Pill, and most without any idea of the harm they could be causing to their bodies.[47]

Off the Pill and Still Can't Get Pregnant? Here's Why

In order to understand why oral contraceptives might cause infertility after you stop taking them, you have to first understand how the Pill works. Birth control pills are made up of synthetic versions of estrogen and progesterone that suppress the body's natural production of progesterone. That's key to how they prevent pregnancy. The synthetic hormones stop the body's natural progesterone from activating and creating a thicker uterine lining each month so that an egg can be fertilized and implanted in that lining. Your brain actually dictates all of this from within the pituitary gland. Follicle-stimulating hormone (FSH) is released in the brain and "tells" the ovary to produce a follicle every month—around day 14, also known as ovulation. At this point, the luteinizing hormone (LH) surge happens; scientists still don't fully understand the whole process, but this surge causes estrogen to rise. When this happens, the follicle is released into your fallopian tube and makes its way to your uterus. But, when you're on birth control, your body eliminates the LH surge, thereby eliminating ovulation completely. Therefore, it's only logical to conclude that OCPs affect the brain, namely the pituitary gland. In fact, at least one study has looked at this possibility and concluded, "OCP use in healthy women is associated with smaller hypothalamic and pituitary volumes, which may be related to disruption of known trophic effects of ovarian sex hormones, although our study design precludes confirmation of any specific mechanism."[48]

As you might imagine, when you take synthetic hormones over a certain period of time, your body can begin to lose the ability to create its own natural progesterone (think: pro-gestation) so that pregnancy can occur.[49] Therefore, though your mind is ready to make a baby, when it comes time to stop taking oral contraception so you can conceive with your partner, your body might not be capable of doing so. Or, even if an egg does get fertilized, your uterine lining might not be able to thicken enough to maintain the pregnancy, resulting in a miscarriage. As I stated before, miscarriage is often related to low progesterone,[50] but many women have no idea that their multiple miscarriages might be caused by it. To put that into perspective, 10 to 20 percent of known pregnancies end in miscarriage,[51] but the percentage is likely higher because so many miscarriages can happen before a woman even knows she is pregnant. On the low end, that's approximately 636,900 miscarriages in the US out of the 6,369,000 pregnancies in a single year. Let's cut that number in half to overly account for the number of those that went unnoticed or were induced (abortion), leaving us with 318,450 women going through the exhausting tragedy of miscarriage. That's 318,450 women overcome with sadness at the realization that the future that had just begun to take shape for them was lost; 318,450 women losing income and some measure of quality of life because of the disruption to their career and/or the cost they may have put into IVF or similar procedures; 318,450 women missing days, weeks, months, even years of their lives because they are picking up the pieces of their broken hope. And that's only a single year, and only in the US.

What to Do Next

If you are questioning whether your past history of oral contraceptives could be the culprit for your current infertility issues, get your hormones analyzed. Most importantly, find a provider who specializes in bioidentical hormone therapy because often a regular doctor will test you and tell you everything is fine. Functional medicine physicians and physicians who specialize in BHRT (bioidentical hormone replacement therapy) use specialized testing that can evaluate your cycle throughout the month and determine if, indeed, your hormones are out of balance. If they are, they can discuss options for bioidentical (not synthetic) progesterone replacement with your OB/Gyn. In a short time and with the right amount of progesterone, you could be holding a baby in your arms. That is my goal for you.

Now, let's say you've never taken birth control in your life, but you are still unable to get pregnant or to maintain a full-term pregnancy. The problem can still be due to low progesterone, and very likely is, based on my experience with thousands of patients. Aside from birth control pills, several aspects of your lifestyle can have a direct impact on your progesterone levels. Sometimes low progesterone can be a result of your gut microbiome being out of balance due to antibiotic use (recent or in the past), poor diet, toxin exposure, and more. Diet is also a huge culprit. Low progesterone could be caused by exposure to environmental estrogens, from either your food or water. Excessive exercise can also cause progesterone and estrogen to drop, so if you're spending hours in the gym, running marathons regularly, or doing any other form of extreme exercise, that could be the problem.

Stress is another big culprit and can cause an imbalance in your hormones, including your progesterone levels. So keep all of these factors in mind as you analyze your health and your fertility. Here's the bottom line: if you are struggling with fertility, no matter what the potential causes, the first order of business is to have your hormones analyzed. You need that data in order to understand what is going on in your body to be able to do something about it.

It's tragic to think how many women have suffered miscarriage after miscarriage, many of whom were never fully evaluated for hormone imbalance, never fully realizing it was related to their hormones, or that there was something easy, affordable, and noninvasive that could be done about it. That's one of the many reasons I feel so passionate about writing this book and getting it into the hands of as many women as possible. You deserve to know the truth and to be empowered by it. I believe that fertility is the birthright of women and you need to understand the many factors at play when optimizing your fertility.

Postpartum Blues / Depression

Postpartum depression (PPD) is another mismanaged issue that plagues women on a regular basis. I have seen many patients for postpartum depression, and here's how the situation often plays out:

A patient, who has recently given birth, comes in: "I feel terrible. I cry all the time. I can't stop. I don't know what's wrong with me. I'm anxious all the time. I am not happy, but I know I'm supposed to be. I just had a baby!"

"You are not alone," I reply. "This is a common postpartum sign of a hormonal imbalance. I've had countless patients just like you. What did your OB/Gyn say?" I asked.

"She offered me an antidepressant, but I don't really want to take one. I mean I've never been depressed in my life."

"I understand," I reply. "Most women feel scared or nervous to even talk about it. There are so many women out there suffering in silence, too afraid to talk to anyone about how they feel because this is supposed to be a joyful time. It's true that the conventional solution for managing postpartum depression is often antidepressants, but you are right in thinking that is not fixing the root cause."

Since starting my medical career and after having my own three children, I find it frustrating the way postpartum depression is addressed in our country. And I think the issue is multifaceted. I had a conversation recently with a woman from Europe who gave birth to her baby in Holland. After the mother went home from the hospital, a nurse came to the house to check on the mother and baby three times daily, every day, for six weeks. I was shocked. Can you imagine how that would change things and how different the postpartum experience would be if we had that kind of care in America? Most of my patients who have had postpartum depression have never had this type of postnatal follow up, and they certainly have never had their hormones discussed or addressed. If they bring them up with their OB/Gyn, they have been told their hormones don't matter. Why would it not make sense that this shift in your hormones is the cause of your mental health decline? Postpartum depression affects one in seven mothers, or four hundred thousand births every year.[52] To the extreme, these women are at a much higher risk for suicide. I have heard stories of women in my own community who have committed suicide because of the incredibly profound depression they experienced postpartum. According to the Statistical Manual of Mental Disorders, PPD is diagnosed when a new mom experiences at least five of the following depressive symptoms for at least two weeks:

- Depressed mood (subjective or observed) is present most of the day

- Loss of interest or pleasure, most of the day

- Insomnia or hypersomnia

- Psychomotor retardation or agitation

- Worthlessness or guilt

- Loss of energy or fatigue

- Suicidal ideation or attempt and recurrent thoughts of death

- Impaired concentration or indecisiveness

- Change in weight or appetite (weight change 5% over 1 month)[53]

I would argue that more than one out of seven women experience at least a few of these symptoms. For those who are screened and determined to be depressed postpartum, only 25 percent receive any kind of follow-up care aside from being prescribed an antidepressant.[54] Their hormones usually go unchecked, which doesn't make sense to me given the dramatic physiological change that birthing a baby brings about. I have had many patients come into my practice, having begged their OB/Gyns to check their hormones because they felt like their postpartum depression was due to hormone imbalance, but their OB/Gyn did not want to do the testing and/or did not know how to interpret the test results.[55]

I'll never forget a patient who came to see me a few months after she had her first baby. She was suffering from postpartum depression and wasn't getting the help she needed. She told me that, prior to seeing me, she asked her OB/Gyn if he would check her hormones. He said no. She then went to another OB/Gyn, who also said no. She went back to her regular OB/Gyn and he relented and said,

"Fine. I will check them, but it won't really matter because there is nothing to be done about it."

When this patient came in to see me, I checked her hormones and found there had been a significant decrease in her progesterone. I prescribed progesterone and, after months of suffering, she finally felt back to herself. You see, when you deliver your baby, your placenta is delivered too. This placenta is rich in progesterone, which is our body's natural happy hormone. So if you don't have enough of a reserve, it can cause you to be deficient. In fact, just a small amount of progesterone cream might be all you need.

The difference in progesterone levels from prepregnancy to pregnancy to postpartum can be substantial. Normal progesterone levels in women prepregnancy can range from less than 1 nanogram per milliliter (ng/mL) to 20 ng/mL. During pregnancy, progesterone levels skyrocket as high as 300 ng/mL. And then progesterone returns to normal or below-normal levels postpartum.[56] I often see women's levels at 0.5 ng/mL postpartum, significantly less than what they were prior to pregnancy. No matter what range you fall in, the dramatic decrease in progesterone after birth can have a substantial impact on mental health.

Why then doesn't every woman experience postpartum depression? It all depends on your progesterone reserve. Some women have enough of a reserve to not notice the deficiency postpartum. Other times, and as is the case with postpartum depression, we don't have enough and now those "baby blues"; or depression; or at the extreme, psychosis, can come into play and we feel crazy (not to mention having difficulty bonding, loss of appetite, fatigue, insomnia, and feelings of shame and guilt). That's how patients like Meredith end up in my office. The reaction from Meredith's doctor was something I've heard again and again from my patients. The "standard of care" for PPD is antidepressants.

We are doing a great disservice to mothers, their newborn babies, and society at large by not treating the root cause. If we can't figure out how to take care of women postpartum, then what are we doing right? Meredith was lucky that she had a friend who was a patient of mine, who recommended she come to me to get a second opinion and to get her hormones checked. I think about the millions of women who feel they have no other choice but to put their faith in their obstetricians. Now don't get me wrong, OB/Gyns are amazing physicians who do everything in their power to care for the health of mother and baby. I wholeheartedly loved my OB/Gyn. But it is important to know that you may very well need another physician to address your mental health postpartum.

Many women don't have the resources to seek a second opinion and have to take their doctor's, and by extension, the pharmaceutical companies', word that their solution for PPD is right. My main goal as a functional medicine physician and mother is to make women aware of, and encourage them to pursue, a different option. Not only are antidepressants not the answer for most women because they don't solve the root problem of hormone imbalance, but there is also extremely limited research on the long-term effects of antidepressants on infants via breast milk. Even if women don't breastfeed, antidepressants are still not the answer. My patient who was prescribed antidepressants while she was breastfeeding did not want her baby impacted, only to find out years later that the antidepressants had detrimental neurological effects. We don't know if that would have been the case, but we don't know for sure that it wouldn't either.

Even before I start to cover more about why antidepressants are most likely the wrong choice, there's a bigger problem at hand: lack of follow up. So you deliver your baby, go home in a few days, and are left to figure things out. You see your pediatrician a couple of days later, who assesses the baby. But what about you? You see your OB/Gyn at the six-week postpartum mark to have a quick check-in, discuss birth control and breastfeeding, and have a short screening about your mood. Do we really think that is enough? You have just gone through a major life event. So, what if you say your mood is poor? You are most likely prescribed a basic antidepressant but never have a conversation about your hormones.

Meanwhile, you continue with the regular trips to the pediatrician where you analyze such questions as: What's the baby's weight? How many times does the baby pee? Poop? How many ounces of milk is he or she taking? The nearly obsessive observation of every minuscule milestone of your child's life begins in the delivery room and continues for years. And that obsession, by the way, is enough to make any woman feel crazy and out of control. It's like she's not the boss of her own baby . . . that she doesn't know what's best for her child . . . that her baby is somehow suffering, not getting enough to eat, not peeing or pooping at regular intervals, not meeting milestones. Whatever happened to maternal instinct?

The messages mothers receive in those early weeks, months, and years are that they aren't capable of knowing what's best for their baby, so they must outsource this knowledge to an army of doctors, nurses, and lactation specialists. This, in turn, can trigger anxiety, insecurity, and self-doubt, which only compounds symptoms of postpartum depression. An ugly cycle, for sure. I'm not saying that these medical providers are not needed; I am saying that our medical system often takes maternal instinct out of the equation. Of course, I'm not implying doctors are intentionally gaslighting mothers or they're just out to make money on prescriptions. I truly believe that most people who feel called to the field of medicine set out with a pure desire to make a difference and to have a positive impact on people's lives.

We know that mother-baby bonding is the most important aspect of the baby's health early on.[57] It's only logical that the physical and mental health of the mom has a direct impact on the health of the baby, so you'd think there would be a heck of a lot more attention paid to it. I firmly believe that the traditional medical system has failed mothers in that there's no provision for someone to sit down with the mom on a regular basis during the first year and sympathetically and warmly approach her about how she's faring. And then listen to her. Give her space to feel safe, to really open up about the emotional roller coaster of motherhood. This doesn't have to be complicated either. In fact, in the next chapter, I'm going to share a simple list of questions that gives us the information we need.

And as I stressed earlier, if the mother is struggling, the knee-jerk answer should not be an antidepressant. Communication and compassion for the mom should come first and, if needed, managing the hormonal imbalance. By treating this imbalance, brain chemistry goes back to normal, and mom can go back to happily bonding with her baby. In my perfect world, that's how it would play out. I wish it would be this way for every mom who is battling postpartum depression. Unfortunately, we are working within what I perceive to be a broken system. The good news is: if you know it's broken, you can find new ways to navigate it.

Navigating Postpartum Depression

In the United States, when you're considering getting pregnant or are already pregnant, one of your first "to dos" is to make sure you have an obstetrician or, less commonly, a midwife you trust. One of the topics you should absolutely be discussing with your doctor is your hormones. If you historically have low progesterone before you get pregnant, then you have a higher risk of experiencing extremely low progesterone after giving birth, which means you are susceptible to postpartum depression. If you have your hormones tested before you get pregnant, you can decrease your risks. Let's dive into the why and how behind all of this.

When your "happy hormone," progesterone, is in proper balance with your other hormones, it helps you sleep, regulates your cycle, balances estrogen, and most importantly, reduces anxiety and depression. Progesterone is produced in the ovaries and, during pregnancy, in the placenta. Therefore, if you went into pregnancy with low progesterone but felt fantastic in the second and third trimesters, that was due to the boost in progesterone that you were getting from the growing placenta. However, when you deliver the baby and the placenta, all that extra progesterone goes with it. This is exactly why it is so crucial to have your hormones assessed before pregnancy and at least be aware that if you have low progesterone, you may develop postpartum depression. It would be smart to have a prescription for progesterone on hand so that you can take it postpregnancy if you feel the baby blues or worse. If it were up to me, I would give every woman a bottle of progesterone immediately after having a baby. Now, do I think every woman would need to take it? No, but it's often the perfect fix for postpartum depression. There are countless women who experience normal mother-baby bonding and never for a moment feel they are dealing with postpartum depression. But for those on the opposite end of the spectrum, or somewhere in between, this would be a miraculous solution.

How *Should* I Feel after Giving Birth?

When I look at the standard list of questions that OBs ask their patients to assess whether they're dealing with PPD, I see basically the same assessment tool used by psychologists and psychiatrists for diagnosing depression but adapted with some questions related to having a baby. But here's the thing: "regular" depression and postpartum depression are not one and the same. They don't share the same root cause, and women don't experience them in the same way. Rather than asking questions that don't really apply, I think we should shift the focus to how you should be feeling overall.

In the first days and weeks after giving birth, you should be feeling elated. It should feel like you're exactly where you are supposed to be. Our bodies are meant to do this; it's how we were created. You're supposed to be feeling an intense bond with your baby. Of course, you'll feel tired and like you've been through a major event, because you have. But you should not be feeling hopeless, isolated, scared to be alone, like a terrible mother, or that you don't want to be with your baby. If you feel these things, you need help. Or if you are disconnecting and feeling separated from your spouse or not finding joy in anything, those are also signs of postpartum depression.

If this is you, then I do not want you to feel ashamed. You have not done anything wrong and it is not your fault. You—all of us—have the capacity to be a wonderful mom. As covered already in this chapter, you likely have a hormone deficiency and need your progesterone boosted. Now, if you are scratching your head and thinking that being a mom is not 100 percent euphoria all the time, but it's also not all dark clouds and desperation, that is perfectly normal. Listen, having a baby, and breastfeeding the baby, is neither easy nor painless. Your uterus is cramping, your breasts hurt, and sometimes you might feel miserable because you just want a break from it all. As I shared in chapter 2, I was lucky in that my OB/Gyn with my first child was very progressive and very honest. She mentally prepared me for the pains of breastfeeding. She also explained that breastfeeding would trigger oxytocin in my brain, which would cause my uterus to contract back down to its normal size, so it wasn't a surprise when I experienced cramps while I was breastfeeding. It all subsided and became much easier in the few weeks following delivery.

I think society ultimately makes women feel like they're doing something wrong all the time. Culture tends to paint a picture of perfection when it comes to having an infant, or children of any age. But no one is perfect, and no one comes out unscathed. Too often we aren't honest enough about the messy parts, the painful parts, of becoming a mom or of being a woman, really. I also think society has taken a wrong turn by putting way too much pressure on the mom. Here you are trying to be strong for the baby, trying to do it all, and you don't have a team to support you. We look to the dad, and it's great if he's able to get up in the middle of the night to assist with feedings or changing diapers, but dad needs to be well-rested too. I had one mom tell me that her husband had to sleep in another part of the house because he was an anesthesiologist, and he needed a certain amount of sleep in order to do his job well. (If you were one of his patients, you'd want him to feel wide awake and focused before he put you under, right?)

Yes, paternity leave is becoming more common in the US, but it's currently a rarity rather than the norm. I believe the standard maternity and paternity leave in America does not allow for enough support for mom when there are so many demands on our time and energy.[58] I know many working women who only took six weeks off for maternity leave because that's all they were afforded by their company, but the bonding period is critical during the first six months. Our society has to change this norm.

When we look at other cultures across the world, they embrace a "village" mentality. A woman gives birth, and other women gather around and help her find her footing. They are there day and night, sharing the work as well as their wisdom and experience. Women in those cultures aren't having to reinvent the wheel each and every time they become a mom. They lean on each other for help and support, and both mom and baby benefit greatly from it.

What's the takeaway for those of us living modern lives in suburban cities and towns? If you have women in your life who are willing to step up and help you in those first weeks, by all means, ask for help. Don't try to be "strong" and do it all alone. Alleviate the stress where you can. If your trusted friend or family member offers to come watch the baby so you can take a nap in the afternoon, take them up on it. I think we need to make a critical shift in our culture toward leaning on one another for support instead of trying to do everything solo. It does not make us "super mom" if we can function on one hour of sleep. It just makes us tired, susceptible to illness, and, over time, resentful. My suggestion is to accept help if it's offered and seek it out if it's not.

Postpartum Quiz—
Treat the Cause, Not the Symptom

When I sit down with a postpartum mom for the first time, and especially if I wasn't treating her before pregnancy and have no history on her, I ask these questions:

1. Did you have heavy periods before you got pregnant?

2. Did you experience PMS symptoms, including mood swings, depression, or anxiety, at specific times in your cycle?

3. How did you feel during your pregnancy after the first trimester? Were you happier than you'd felt in a long time?

Once we've covered those bases and have had a discussion about what she should be feeling and experiencing, if it's obvious she's having the opposite experience, then the path forward is very clear. If she's suffering, I treat her with progesterone. Period. Do not waste time on a hormone test. The risk of postpartum depression is too great to delay treatment. Take progesterone that night, before bed.

Luckily, it's very affordable and accessible. It comes in the form of a capsule or a cream. The effect is incredible, and every time I take that course of action, the mom calls me a few days or a week later thanking me for turning it all around.

I know it sounds simple. And really, it often is. What I've learned after practicing medicine for as long as I have is that the medical community tends to overcomplicate things. Let's remember Occam's razor: "The simplest solution is almost always the best." The root cause of postpartum depression hormone imbalance is usually low progesterone. When we get the progesterone levels back up, depression disappears. No one outside of functional medicine is talking about PPD this way. All the focus has been on the symptom: depression. But we should always treat the root cause, not the symptom.

An Intravenous Drug for PPD?

A few years ago, the FDA approved a drug to treat postpartum depression that costs between $20,000 and $30,000. It's called Zulresso (brexanolone), and it was the first of its kind approved by the FDA specifically for PPD.[59]

While you might think the price tag is the worst part, in my opinion, it's not. This treatment is comprised of a sixty-hour IV drug that postpartum women must go to the hospital to receive, which means time away from their newborn baby during a critical time of bonding.[60] After three days away from the baby, returning to breast-feeding again can be really challenging. Even if mom pumps her milk during that stint in the hospital, her milk volume will have decreased and she will have missed out on those opportunities for her brain to release oxytocin while nursing, which in turn improves mental health.

Plus, the treatment carries with it a long list of potential side effects, as the Mayo Clinic website warns: "This medicine may cause some people to be agitated, irritable, or display other abnormal behaviors. It may also cause some people to have suicidal thoughts and tendencies or to become more depressed." [61] I understand that women suffering with PPD can feel desperate and terrified, so I can see why they might be willing to do anything. But still, this drug carries serious potential side effects, is incredibly costly, and breaks down the mother-baby bond. The answer can be very simple—bioidentical progesterone can make the difference, without all the risks.

I do want to note: Since the drug first came out, the FDA did approve it in an oral form.[62] So, that's an improvement over going to the hospital for a sixty-hour infusion. But it's still not addressing the root cause from a simple and cost-effective perspective.

My message to you is this: If your medical provider recommends a "treatment" for PPD that takes you away from your baby and puts you in a hospital for three days, consider what you've learned in this book and that there might be an alternative solution.

More Postpartum Tips

Bringing a child into the world is tough, not only on mom but on a family unit. Especially if help isn't readily available, your life can be turned upside down by the arrival of a baby. As a physician, my primary focus is on how you can get your body into equilibrium, especially as it relates to your hormones but outside the body as well. This is why I want to share with you some insight into how you can make the tough times less difficult so you can be fully present and really experience the joy-filled moments, the hilariously ridiculous moments, and the peaceful, quiet moments too. Your whole environment, your relationships, your home, your routine—all of it plays into how you feel. I like to help my patients think this way so that they can really program their lifestyle for success. The days, weeks, and months following the birth of a child can actually be (mostly) wonderful if you prepare your mind, body, home, and relationships in realistic ways. Here are some tips:

Take sleep seriously. Sleep helps regulate your hormones. When you're sleep deprived and your circadian rhythms are out of whack, you can end up experiencing what's called a "hormone cascade." This has a detrimental effect on both men and women, so this isn't advice limited to moms alone. I often see men with newborns at home experiencing really low testosterone and high cortisol. That's because men make testosterone, estradiol, and cortisol out of pregnenolone and, without proper sleep, the body gets stressed and goes into fight-or-flight mode, which means it shifts to produce more cortisol and less testosterone. It's imperative that men do what they can to decrease cortisol production, and the simplest fix is to get serious about sleep.

The same goes for women. When women are consistently sleep deprived, their cortisol production also goes up, testosterone goes down, and progesterone can also be negatively impacted. When hormones become dysregulated as a result of sleep deprivation, cravings for carbohydrates kick in because hunger hormones are out of balance; and the immune system takes a big hit. This is also when we can develop dependencies on alcohol or sleeping drugs, which cause the cascade to continue. Lack of sleep also puts us at even greater risk for depression. One thing leads to another, and before we know it, we're sick, tired, moody, and gaining weight, and it all stems from not taking sleep seriously. If you do nothing else when you have a newborn at home, focus on cracking the code on your good night's sleep.

I know how tough it is to practice any kind of normal sleep routine when you have a newborn. As I covered in chapter 2, this will likely go against most of what you've heard regarding sleeping with your baby, but for me, co-sleeping was the answer. I can honestly say I never felt sleep deprived thanks to the fact that I slept with my baby tucked into my arm for the first year. And mind you, I was still in residency when I had my first two babies. Co-sleeping is very natural—at least for the first six months of life—because your baby is wired to want to be right next to you. That is where the baby is safest; you are the baby's lifeline and food supply.

Historically, cultural and biological anthropology tells us the same: all mammals, primates, and the majority of non-Western societies co-sleep. American society, however, encourages us to have the baby sleep in its own room—the nursery. That idea truly goes against how humans and most animals are wired. Co-sleeping is a form of natural and healthy regulation between parent and baby: you regulate each other's brain waves, REM cycles, oxygen levels, and even breathing.[63] The skin-to-skin contact is healthy and contributes to bonding, and the regulation supports synaptogenesis—the growth and new connections between neurons in newborns.[64] Additionally, in studies comparing babies who co-slept and those who slept separately (both human and primate), even when the baby sleeping separately adjusts after a few nights, their cortisol (stress) levels remain high compared to the co-sleeping baby.[65]

Clearly, you want to be careful with co-sleeping. If you or your partner is an extraordinarily deep sleeper, overweight, a very active sleeper, or you are just terrified that you will roll over on your baby, do not consider co-sleeping. If you cannot co-sleep, I recommend that you have the baby's bassinet near your bed, so you are not getting up multiple times a night and trudging to the nursery. You'll be able to get back to sleep quicker after a feeding if the baby is right there in your bedroom with you. I encourage you to prioritize your sleep and figure out a routine that truly works for your family. Your hormones and your health will thank you.

Make Exercise a Priority. Exercise and good sleep go hand in hand. Even if you're feeling exhausted, creating a realistic daily exercise routine is crucial. It will help you fall asleep at night, it will reduce stress, and it will help your body secrete "happy hormones" to help you with mood regulation. Don't set the bar too high for exercise. Instead, find a way to move your body that doesn't completely wear you out but instead leaves you feeling energized. If you worked out regularly before the baby, realize that you may need to adjust your normal routine to give your body time to fully heal and get back into the swing of things. If you had to go on bed rest or you were not able to work out as much as you usually do during pregnancy, now is the time to create a new routine.

I loved yoga before, during, and after pregnancy. It served me well with all three of my deliveries, as well as in postpartum healing. I did the hardest classes available at the yoga studio I attended, not the yoga-for-pregnancy classes. I was the only pregnant woman in my classes and I did them up until the final weeks of pregnancy. Doing this was amazing for my body and kept me fit and strong. I recommend finding something that will help you work up a sweat and keep you fit. Yoga may not be your thing, but maybe swimming, jogging, or biking is. Just don't allow yourself to slip into a daily routine that doesn't include regular movement.

Our bodies are made to move; it's when we become sedentary that problems arise. Regular exercise applies to both mom and dad. Men, your hormones also need you to get up and move that body. Prevent a hormonal cascade by including cardiovascular exercise as well as resistance training, proper stretching, and regular breath work in your routine.

Take Your Postpartum Health into Your Own Hands

I hope by now you're starting to realize that you cannot outsource your postpartum wellness to your obstetrician or midwife. They are wholly focused on helping you safely deliver your baby, which is wonderful, but that's often where their involvement ends. Other than a quick visit at six weeks postdelivery, you generally cannot rely on them to be involved in your health going forward, especially where your hormones are concerned.

That's why I want to empower you to take your postpartum health into your own hands. Take steps to prioritize your overall health by incorporating the tips I've shared with you and by listening and responding to the needs of your own body. If you aren't feeling like yourself, or you're dealing with emotional upheaval, seek the advice of a functional medicine doctor or another physician you trust to really listen to your concerns and not just quickly prescribe an antidepressant and send you on your way.

Make it clear that you are looking for another answer and you want to understand what's going on in your body and with your hormones. Knowledge is power. The more time you invest in learning about how your hormones work and knowing the signs when they might be unbalanced, the less time you'll have to spend feeling unhappy, frustrated, or like you aren't able to fully enjoy being a mom. It does not have to be a mystery, and you do not have to be miserable. Take the reins on your physical and mental health today. You (and your baby) will be so glad you did.

Dr. Taylor's Checklist
for Your Thirties

1. Pregnancy and infertility: Consider your hormones if you can't get pregnant or stay pregnant. Appropriate levels of progesterone are vital to avoiding miscarriage. Diet, stress, and your gut health are all important to address as well.

2. Postpartum depression: Low progesterone is a key factor in postpartum depression. If you are concerned about your risk for postpartum depression, make sure you are seeking out the help of a functional medicine provider or OB/Gyn who will prescribe progesterone postpartum. This can be a lifesaver.

3. Parenthood:

   • Figure out a sleeping arrangement that allows for you and your partner to get as much solid sleep per night as possible.

   • Connect with your baby, and lean into the "village" of people in your life who can help you really have quality bonding time with your child.

- Prioritize daily exercise that you enjoy. Moving your body is critical during this time.

- Choose foods that nourish your body and your baby's body while breastfeeding.

Chapter 6

YOUR FORTIES

So, you are in your forties. You may have had kids and now you're busy raising them, working, and managing a full life. As I've seen in many patients, your own health and happiness might have migrated down to the bottom of your list of priorities. You likely don't have the energy you did in your twenties. This is the age when libido begins to plummet. Sleep quality starts to decline. And you might just feel like this is your new normal as you age. But your hormones are also changing, and this affects how you feel every day. Let's first look at testosterone, because this is the first hormone to fall as you approach menopause, and this decline often happens in your early forties.

In your forties, your periods start to change, possibly becoming less frequent, especially in your late forties. This is the time in life when people are often diagnosed with chronic diseases like high blood pressure, type 2 diabetes, and high cholesterol. The first go-to solution should not be medication. Functional medicine can be crucial for evaluating the key causes for these chronic diseases. As with each decade, focusing on a healthy diet filled with lots of fruits and vegetables, prioritizing sleep, and exercising frequently is important. I also think managing stress is key. Are you constantly running around taking your kids here and there? Are you struggling to find time to decompress? All these things affect your overall health.

If you have high blood pressure, start with lifestyle changes. Incorporate deep-breathing exercises every day for at least thirty minutes. A study that looked at twenty research articles found that "slow breathing can be used as an alternate, non-pharmacological therapy for hypertension individuals to reduce blood pressure."[66] Supplements like magnesium can also be super helpful for lowering blood pressure. For blood sugar control, a supplement called berberine can be very helpful because it can reduce glucose levels.[67] For cholesterol, I love plant sterols and bergamot. The combination can be incredible for reducing cholesterol.

As I mentioned, our forties are when testosterone starts to decline. Testosterone can be an incredibly powerful tool in your overall wellness toolbox. Women are often surprised they need it because it's generally thought of as a male hormone. As soon as I supplement a woman's testosterone, they often feel a massive shift not only in libido but in motivation, drive, energy, and duration of and recovery from workouts. It can be a game changer. So if your sex drive isn't what it used to be, get your testosterone checked by a bioidentical hormone replacement therapy (BHRT) expert. I have seen lives changed with testosterone therapy. Moreover, when couples both take it, it makes a huge difference in their relationship.

Testosterone treatments for men have been FDA approved for decades, but despite evidence of efficacy and safety, the FDA has yet to approve them for women in the United States. According to a 2012 study published in the *Journal of Sexual*

Medicine, transdermal testosterone appears to be an effective and safe therapy for postmenopausal women with hypoactive sexual desire disorder (HSDD).[68] Furthermore, in a 2016 study published in the journal *Fertility and Sterility,* researchers concluded that "the use of transdermal T is associated with an increase in androgenic adverse events such as acne but is not associated with any serious adverse events."[69] In a paper published in 2022 by Dr. Gary Donovitz, he states:

> According to Panay and Fenton, young women's ovaries produce approximately three to four times more testosterone than estrogen daily. In 2002, Dimitrakakis et al. stated that testosterone is the most abundant biologically active gonadal hormone throughout the female lifespan. However, unfortunately, due to a plethora of misconceptions, women remain without any FDA-approved testosterone therapies, while more than 30 approved testosterone therapies are available for men. This has

resulted in millions of women suffering in silence with very common symptoms that could easily be addressed with the use of testosterone.[70]

These symptoms are exactly what I treat in my office. So how do you know if you need testosterone treatment? The signs and symptoms of androgen insufficiency (low testosterone) in women include a diminished sense of well-being, low libido, decreased drive and motivation, and low muscle mass. I can't tell you how many women come into my office with exactly these symptoms. And when their testosterone is optimized, they feel like a different person.

Let's get back to the concept that testosterone is viewed as a male hormone and doesn't play a significant role in women's bodies. After all, it's common to hear about men suffering from "low T," but we don't hear anyone talking about women having the same issue. When have you ever seen commercials, billboards, or magazine ads for testosterone treatments for women? But testosterone is so important for a woman's well-being, and it is "the most important circulating and naturally occurring androgen in both men and women. In women, testosterone is produced primarily through peripheral conversion of androstenedione (50 percent) with the remainder of production concentrated in the ovary (25 percent) and adrenal cortex (25 percent)."[71]

Testosterone is the most abundant active steroid in women, with its levels being even higher than estradiol levels.[72] And in the same way that testosterone gradually decreases over time in men, testosterone also decreases over time in women.[73]

You might be wondering if testosterone treatments could cause you to have "roid rage" or experience increased agitation or aggression. That's another common misconception. If your testosterone becomes too high, you can experience increased irritability, but if you are being managed by a BHRT specialist and your levels are monitored, then you should not experience these symptoms.

I prescribe all forms of bioidentical testosterone for women, but I find that one of the most effective treatments for my peri- and menopausal patients is pellet therapy. I had never heard of pellet therapy prior to starting my practice, but after about a year of seeing patients, I had patients asking me if I prescribed them. Just to explain a bit, pellets are compounded testosterone and/or estradiol that are inserted underneath the skin to provide a consistent release of hormones into the system over a three-to-four-month period. Your doctor implants the pellets just underneath your skin in the lower hip/buttock region. The hormones are released into your system based on your cardiac output, so as you are up and moving around, your heart is pumping harder and the blood supply that has grown around the pellets is extracting hormones from the pellets and pulling them into your bloodstream. Therefore, the more active you are, the better.

So I did a lot of research after my patients continued to ask me about them and started performing the procedure in 2016. Since then, I have done thousands of procedures and my patients find them to be life-changing. It's an incredible form of balancing hormones. I don't recommend them for everybody, but for the patients I do pellet, the difference in overall health and wellness is astonishing.

History and Success of Testosterone Replacement in Women

Believe it or not, subcutaneous testosterone therapy delivered by pellet implantation has been used with success in female patients since 1938.[74] Published data demonstrates efficacy as well as safety in doses of 75 mg up to 225 mg. And even higher doses (500–1800 mg) of subcutaneous testosterone have been safely used, specifically to treat breast cancer patients.[75] This is not a new concept.

In a 2010 study published in the journal *Maturitas*, researchers set out to measure the effectiveness of continuous testosterone therapy in three hundred pre- and postmenopausal women. Before they were treated, study participants were asked to fill out a questionnaire[76] in order to identify the type and severity of symptoms they were experiencing. It asked questions about hot flashes, sweating, heart discomfort, sleep problems, anxiety, exhaustion, sexual issues, vaginal dryness, joint pain, and more.

Then patients received the testosterone treatment delivered by subcutaneous implant for three months, after which they filled out the questionnaire again to determine whether they experienced any improvement. The women experienced a marked improvement in all eleven categories, even after just three months of treatment. The authors of the study wrote in conclusion, "This study has shown for the first time that adequate doses of continuous testosterone alone, delivered by subcutaneous implant, was effective therapy for physical, psychological, and urogenital symptoms in both pre- and post-menopausal women, suggesting a broader physiologic role for testosterone. Despite methodological limitations, our clinical observations along with existing data support the concept that testosterone administration improves quality of life."[77]

If you haven't considered testosterone replacement therapy before, I hope this chapter has convinced you to investigate it further. I know it can be intimidating to try something that isn't technically FDA approved, but I would encourage you to think beyond what you have traditionally been taught. If something resonates, especially if there is data to back it up (as in the case of testosterone replacement), it's worth exploring.

Dr. Taylor's Checklist for Your Forties:

- Get your hormones evaluated by a functional medicine physician.

- Take berberine for improved blood sugar control and to decrease insulin resistance.

- Keep your weight at a healthy level, and aim for a waist-to-hip ratio of 0.85 or less.

- Exercise regularly; again, it's important to identify an exercise routine that you enjoy and that is realistic for your schedule and lifestyle.

- Properly manage your stress and keep yourself high on your list of priorities.

- Don't let your libido determine your relationship. Your low sex drive might have nothing to do with your partner and may have everything to do with your testosterone. Have a discussion with your BHRT provider and consider testosterone replacement therapy.

- If your blood pressure is increasing, try yoga, deep-breathing exercises, and supplementing with magnesium.

- If your cholesterol is increasing, try eliminating dairy (e.g., cream in your coffee) and eggs and increase your fiber and vegetable intake. If necessary, start supplementing with plant sterols and bergamot.

- If you are married, be intentional about connecting with your spouse. Plan times for the two of you to get away from your everyday routine.

- If you are feeling depressed, get your hormones checked. Just because your periods are normal does not mean your hormones are optimal.

Chapter 7

YOUR FIFTIES

Menopause is, by far, the number one reason women in their late forties and early fifties start asking questions about their hormones. It's often a new realization that their symptoms are a result of a hormonal imbalance. For many of my patients, it's the first time they have ever dealt with anxiety or depression. And for some, they may experience thoughts of suicide that they had never, ever experienced before. They may have never even experienced PMS or postpartum depression. They may have slept perfectly their whole life, and now all of a sudden, things have changed, and they are not sure why. It can be hard for some women to suspect their hormones are to blame because they may continue to have normal periods and don't have hot flashes (which they know is a telltale sign of menopause). But symptoms vary widely. They may go to their gynecologist, who tells them that their hormones are normal and that they are not in menopause until they haven't had a period for a full year.

I see a very different scenario in my clinic. I see women who have had "normal" periods but are now in "perimenopause" (the onset of menopause, when your body is transitioning from reproductive years into menopause). Their progesterone has decreased, which is affecting their mood and causing anxiety or depression or both. They are also noticing that their hair is falling out, also caused by lower progesterone. They find that their memory isn't as good as usual and they are having a hard time remembering words, another sign of low progesterone. They notice their libido is low and they never really want to have sex anymore, a sign of low testosterone. Maybe you can relate. You may have had your hormones checked and been told everything is normal. That doesn't mean they are normal for *you*.

By now you know I have devoted my medical

career to helping women (and men) get to the root of their hormone problems by treating hormonal deficiencies. For the last decade, I have treated thousands of patients, many of whom were not receiving the care they desperately needed. The typical menopause journey for most women begins with specific symptoms and a trip to the OB/Gyn. For many women, this is the only doctor they see, and they expect their OB/Gyn to have the answers. Often an OB/Gyn will check their hormones and tell their patients that they are "within range."

Let's look at that "range" for a second. Depending on which lab test result is being analyzed, some reference ranges can't be trusted. For example, estradiol that is 15 pg/mL on a lab result is considered "normal" from a conventional perspective, but it is not optimal, even though the lab technically labels your result as being within range. Similarly, progesterone that is 0.5 ng/mL is not optimal, even though the lab says you are within range. For testosterone, there is no defined acceptable range for women. The range is a clinical analysis, meaning the acceptable level of testosterone actually depends on how you feel and what is right for your unique body. While on this reference-range topic, I'd like to add, allopathic medicine practitioners typically rely heavily on how the various laboratories define "normal," based on population samplings. But in functional medicine, we take the whole patient into account, and the lab results are just part of that overall picture. In fact, functional medicine practitioners conduct very different and specialized lab tests than allopathic doctors do, so I often have patients tell me we're doing tests that no other doctor ever conducted. And that gives me the data I need in order to discover the root cause of the patient's symptoms.

Follicle-stimulating hormone (FSH) is another important hormone. Levels over 23 are considered menopausal, which means your hormones (estrogen and progesterone) are very low. I've had patients in their thirties who are in premature menopause, confirmed by a FSH test. Yet so often, women have their labs drawn to check their hormones and find that the results fall "within range" as defined by the lab, and thus conclude that their hormones are not the problem, even if they're experiencing symptoms.

By now you know you can look at your results with a different lens. You understand that while the hormone levels may be "within range," these levels are not necessarily where women feel their best, and artificial ranges should not define your optimum potential. The more you understand your hormones and your levels, the better you will be able to make educated decisions about your health.

Okay, so back to a perimenopausal or menopausal woman's typical journey. You go to your OB/Gyn and expect them to have the answers about your hormones. After all, why wouldn't they? They are the doctor who specifically treats female issues. But they check your hormones and tell you your levels are within range. Now you know not to necessarily trust that. And, again, it's important to recognize that, for the most part, OB/Gyns aren't fully trained to treat menopause and address estrogen, progesterone, and testosterone deficiencies. They lack the training, and therefore, *you* lack the knowledge. So you take the meds they prescribe. After all, what else is there to do? But the meds they prescribe cause you to gain weight and experience a decrease in your libido. You are left feeling numb. And your marriage is suffering. You don't really *want* to be on all these medications, but it seems as though you have no other choices.

As you are probably realizing, the body cannot be treated in parts; it must be treated as a whole because every system is connected, and every system is affected by the others. In my functional medicine practice, I treat the whole body. I have been able to transition numerous patients off antidepressants, antianxiety meds, and sleep meds. And not surprisingly, they feel like a whole new person—often better than they have in decades.

Just imagine being in menopause but having more energy and feeling more vibrant than you did in your thirties. It's possible. I witness it every day. Over time, numerous myths about menopause and hormone replacement therapy have been perpetuated. Unfortunately, when we hear something enough times, we automatically believe it's true. This is why I want to open your eyes to the truth behind menopause, and show you that you can feel vibrant, healthy, and strong as you age.

Quick Q&A

Here are the questions I ask every patient who is either in menopause or approaching it. If this is the stage of life you're currently in, take a moment to answer these questions:

1. Has your mood declined?

   Yes

   No

2. Has your energy declined?

   Yes

   No

3. Are you sleeping through the night?

   Yes

   No

4. Are waking up in the middle of the night unable to go back to sleep?

   Yes

   No

5. Are you waking up with night sweats?

Yes

No

6. Are you having hot flashes?

Yes

No

7. Have you noticed changes in your hair or skin?

Yes

No

8. Are you wondering why you're not feeling yourself?

Yes

No

9. Are you feeling irritable?

Yes

No

10. Has your libido declined?

Yes

No

Now, review your answers. Did you know that no matter what age or stage of life you're in, you don't need to live with *any* of these uncomfortable symptoms? Even if you are in menopause, you don't have to experience hot flashes, night sweats, irritability, lack of libido, poor sleep, or anything else. Right now, let's take a look at the most common menopause myths and the truth about each of them.

Menopause Myth 1: In Order to Be in Menopause, You Must Be Having Hot Flashes

For some of you, menopause hits you like a ton of bricks. Seemingly overnight, you might start experiencing intense night sweats and hot flashes all day long. These are the most well-known symptoms of menopause, so women who experience them usually know it's hormonal and they seek help. For the rest of you, however, it's a slow decline and symptoms begin creeping in during your late thirties or forties, including:

- Difficulty falling asleep and staying asleep

- Feeling anxious or panicky

- Feeling depressed, maybe even suicidal

- Feeling irritable, snapping at their kids or spouse

- Foggy thinking or unable to think of words

- Dry or sagging skin

- Weight gain or difficulty losing weight

- Low libido and inability to orgasm

- And, yes, hot flashes and night sweats

Symptoms can accumulate slowly in a quiet progression of menopause until suddenly you realize that you feel really terrible most of the time, and then you seek out your doctor. Understanding the quietness of menopause is key. It can infiltrate your life without your conscious awareness, but if you're cognizant of what's happening, then you can get what you need to reverse the train. I've seen very dramatic menopausal cases—women in their forties or fifties who were never depressed in their lives but are now experiencing suicidal thoughts. I test their hormones and find they have very low estrogen and progesterone. I put them on hormones and when they come back to see me four weeks later, they feel like a different person. I've also seen women experiencing a slow menopause progression who realize they just aren't themselves. With hormone treatment, they can thrive again.

Here's the truth: menopause is so much more than just hot flashes. In fact, here's how declining hormones affect different parts of the body:

Brain: We have estrogen receptors in our brain, so when our estrogen declines, it leads to cognitive decline and dementia.[78]

Bones: Estrogen is important for maintaining cartilage and protecting joints. The fifties is a time when many women are diagnosed with arthritis. In my practice, I see these symptoms resolve when estrogen is balanced.

Heart: Heart disease is the number one killer of men and women.[79] According to the American Heart Association, "Taking an estrogen pill early in menopause could slow the progress of fatty buildups in the neck arteries, according to new research."[80] Even though there aren't any long-term, prospective studies that specifically examine the use of human bioidentical hormones in menopausal women, there is a substantial amount of research involving estradiol (E2) and progesterone (P4) and how their absence impacts cardiovascular health. The findings strongly indicate that these hormones, when taken together, promote overall female well-being, and particular benefits for the heart and blood vessels have also been seen.[81]

Skin: Estrogen is important for maintaining collagen. Dry and flaky skin is a sign of low estrogen. Vaginal dryness is also a common symptom.

Bladder: Bladder incontinence and frequent urination are common symptoms of menopause. Estrogen provides an antimicrobial barrier, thus preventing UTIs, so when estrogen plummets, women are more susceptible to UTIs and bladder irritation.

Eyes: Estrogen is important for keeping eyes lubricated and avoiding dry eyes.

Menopause Myth 2: Your Primary Doctor or Gynecologist Can Treat Your Hormonal Issues

Would you call an electrician if you needed help with your plumbing? Would you call for an ambulance if your house were burning down? Would a heart doctor operate on your brain? Sure, they all might be able to help, but not in the way you need. Similarly, your primary doctor or gynecologist may not have the training to treat your specific hormone imbalance, read the lab reports correctly, and provide the right treatment. They might provide some treatment, but it likely isn't the best treatment. Even psychiatrists rarely, if ever, look to hormones as the cause, even though they deal with depression and anxiety on a regular basis. Rather than checking a patient's hormones, they'll often start with a low-dose antidepressant or antianxiety medication. Again, those medications treat symptoms, not causes.

Getting your hormones properly evaluated should be the first thing you do when you're experiencing anxiety and depression. That should be the norm in medicine, but until it is, *you* must be your own advocate in searching out quality hormonal care that recognizes and understands the full picture. Your hormones have a deep connection to your mental state, your sleep, your vitality, your libido, and beyond. Without knowing if you have a hormonal imbalance, many doctors are treating you without the information they need to address the underlying issue instead of the symptoms. Depression is a symptom. But for many people, it is not a chemical imbalance; it is a hormonal imbalance. Here's the truth: your doctor may not know how to treat menopause in the most effective way.

Menopause Myth 3: Estrogen Is the *Only* Hormone That Matters

Many people equate "hormones" with "estrogen." Estrogen is traditionally considered the female hormone, and testosterone the male hormone. We tend to think that women have estrogen, men have testosterone, and that's it. Using that logic, many people believe that if a woman is having hormonal issues, then it must be related to estrogen. That's not the whole truth. As Rebecca Glaser and Constantine Dimitrakakis wrote in their article "Testosterone Therapy in Women: Myths and Misconceptions," "Even in scientific publications, testosterone has been referred to as the 'male hormone.' Men do have higher levels of testosterone than women; however, quantitatively, testosterone is the most abundant, active sex steroid in women throughout the female lifespan."[82]

Here's the bottom line: men and women have all the sex hormones—estrogen, progesterone, and testosterone. All three exist in a different balance in each person. To give you a better grasp of the importance of the three key hormones, let's take a closer look at each one:

- Progesterone is our natural antidepressant. In fact, as I stated earlier in the book, postpartum depression can occur as a result of the low progesterone that results after delivery. When you think about mood swings related to PMS, these occur because progesterone is too low. Even though progesterone is a very important and powerful hormone, it simply isn't on people's radar. I will tell you that balancing low progesterone in menopause patients makes the biggest difference—particularly when it comes to optimizing sleep and significantly decreasing or eliminating depression and anxiety.

- Testosterone is about feeling strong, confident, motivated; having a healthy libido; and feeling the vitality we all want as we age. It affects muscle mass, fat distribution, and the ability to lose weight. As we discussed in the previous chapter, there is actually no FDA-approved testosterone treatment for women because the FDA doesn't believe we need it. But women do produce testosterone, and if you produce testosterone, you can also become deficient in it.[83] And as you now know, compared with progesterone and estrogen, testosterone is the most abundant hormone found in women.

Here's the truth: There's much more to look for in hormone testing than just estrogen.

Menopause Myth 4:
This Is Just My Life Now

Maybe you've heard statements like these from well-meaning family, friends, or even your doctor: "Well, this is just how it is when you're in menopause. You just have to grin and bear it. It's all just a normal part of aging. Every woman goes through it."

In America, we tend to value youth and look down on people as they grow older, especially women, as it relates to beauty standards and career. Many physicians don't have good tools and resources for helping people as they age. But did you know that age doesn't have to be one long decline? On the contrary, you can age like a fine wine, growing better with each passing year. Yet how many older people in America do you know who are on dozens of medications? Think about how often you see commercials for prescription medications. Through the influence of Big Pharma, in the US, both doctors and patients have become overly focused on treating the symptoms with meds rather than looking at root causes.

We have seen by now that hormones affect

every part of our body—heart, brain, bones, bladder, joints, skin, eyes. Think about all the many medications that are out there to treat each ailment in these categories. Imagine if we just balanced a menopausal woman's hormones first. We would undoubtedly save her a lifetime of multiple medications for each ache and symptom.

Here's the truth: You can treat the root cause and feel better than you have in decades and save yourself from a lifetime of too many medications.

Menopause Myth 5: Your Doctor Knows What Tests to Do and How to Read Them

Your doctor may request certain lab work, then look at your results and say you are okay, when you know you are not. I've even seen patients who asked their doctor to test them for hormonal issues, and the doctor wouldn't. Or they did a hormone panel, but then they didn't know how to read the results. Here are some lab tests and the results your doctor may not be looking for:

- FSH: A key indicator that the typical doctor is unlikely to look for is your FSH (follicle-stimulating hormone). If this is over 23, you are in menopause and your estrogen is low.

- Progesterone and estrogen: If your progesterone is less than 0.5 ng/mL or your estradiol is less than 15 pg/mL, your hormones are very low and more than likely need to be adjusted.

- Testosterone: Testosterone levels are a little more variable for women, but if your libido is low, then you would more than likely benefit from more testosterone. As I mentioned in chapter 6, I have patients who are on testosterone alone and feel a world of difference. They have a sex life again when before they just accepted that it was a thing of the past. They also have more energy, are self-assured, and feel stronger in general.

Here's the truth: Your doctor may not know what to test for, or how to interpret your results to give you the best treatment plan. So if your numbers and symptoms show that you should pursue treatment, what should that treatment look like? Read on . . .

Menopause Myth 6: All Hormone Treatments Are the Same

You need to know about the differences between *bioidentical* hormones and *synthetic* hormones, and why a compounding pharmacy is your best choice for your hormone regimen. You always want to seek out bioidentical hormones. Here's why (and this is key): Hormones that are found in birth control pills and commonly prescribed menopausal treatments such as Premarin and Prempro, which are made with synthetic estrogen and/or synthetic progesterone. In most cases, the estrogen is made from a pregnant horse's urine (ponder that one for a second). Female horses make twelve different estrogens while female humans make only three (estradiol, estriol, and estrone), so when you ingest synthetic estrogen, your body doesn't recognize it as a self-hormone; it is a foreign substance from an animal. However, bioidentical estrogen, which is derived from plant substances such as yams and soy, is directly identical to the hormones you make. The chemical structure is the same, so your body recognizes it as its own and metabolizes it as you would your own estrogen.

When the Women's Health Initiative came out in 2002 showing that estrogen and progesterone caused strokes, heart attacks, and breast cancer, it was referring to synthetic hormones,[84] not bioidentical. Unfortunately, in the minds of clinicians and patients, all hormone replacement therapy was considered bad. However, in the functional medicine world we believe that bioidentical hormones (in the right amounts) are protective against breast cancer, heart disease (including strokes and heart attacks) and cognitive decline. As I mentioned, our body recognizes them as a self-hormone and knows how to process, use, and metabolize these hormones just as your own body does.

While there are some FDA-approved bioidentical hormones available at your standard pharmacy, most bioidentical hormones are only available at a compounding pharmacy. A compounding pharmacy is able to make hormones specifically for you, and they have a lot more options available than your standard pharmacy. They can make hormones for women and men outside of those that are commercially available. For example, I often prescribe progesterone that is "sustained release," which helps women to fall asleep and stay asleep, a major issue for most menopausal women. That version of progesterone is not commercially available, so I prescribe it through my local compounding pharmacy.

How do you know if your prescribed hormones are bioidentical or synthetic? If it says *progesterone* or *estradiol* or *estriol*, it is bioidentical. If it says *medroxy-progesterone, synthetic progestin,* or *norethindrone*, it is synthetic progesterone. If it says *ethinyl estradiol, estradiol valerate, estropipate, conjugate esterified estrogen*, or *quinestrol*, it is synthetic estrogen. In sum: you want to use bioidentical hormones that have been custom-made for you by a compounding pharmacy under the direction of a doctor who understands bioidentical hormones and how to monitor them.

Here's the truth: there is a vast difference between the types of hormone treatments available to you. Always go with bioidentical, never synthetic.

Menopause Myth 7: All Doctors Are Trained to Treat Hormonal Issues

How do you find the right doctor to help diagnose and treat your hormonal imbalance? If you feel your hormones are off and you mention it to your doctor only to have them shrug it off or tell you to just deal with it, then it's time to find a bioidentical hormone specialist. In my experience, and what I know about how we are trained as physicians, most doctors are not adequately educated to treat hormone imbalances related to PMS, menopause, or andropause (the male version of menopause). It's simply not part of standard medical training in the US. You need to find a functional medicine physician and/or someone who specializes in bioidentical hormones to be treated appropriately. The right treatment is unique to each patient. There is no one-size-fits-all when it comes to hormones. Your symptoms matter; your lab results matter and need to be read correctly too. You want a doctor who really looks at the whole human and how you're feeling. Someone who cares about putting the puzzle pieces together to adequately address the root cause of what you are experiencing.

Now you understand the difference and can research and find a doctor who knows about this healthier way of treating the whole person.

Here's the truth: you can find a doctor who cares about the whole of you and understands hormones in depth too.

If you've been suffering with debilitating symptoms of menopause, I want you to know this: you do not have to live the way you've been living. You don't have to feel the way you're feeling. It is not something you just have to accept as your new normal. You've probably heard the opposite from friends, doctors, your mom or grandma—that you just have to get through it. It's part of life. But it can be done with ease and grace and it can actually be a very smooth transition. There are tools to help you live a high quality of life and make you feel vibrant and energetic as you age. Life is short. Feel your best.

Dr. Taylor's Checklist for Your Fifties

- Get your hormones evaluated by a bioidentical hormone physician or functional medicine physician if you are having any of the symptoms mentioned in this chapter.

  Make sure you are seeing someone who specializes in bioidentical hormones. Your regular doctor may not know how to analyze or treat your hormones.

- Focus on your sleep. Get good quality sleep; don't let this slide.

- Progesterone is a game changer for mood, anxiety, and sleep, especially during this decade.

- Estrogen declines in our late forties or early fifties. Hot flashes and night sweats can occur, but this is also the time when women experience joint pain, bladder issues, and vaginal dryness. Estrogen decline also increases your risk for heart disease, cognitive decline, and bone loss. Low doses of estradiol, either as a patch, a cream, or a pellet, can be super helpful.

- Testosterone is key as you age and is important for maintaining strength and vitality.

Chapter 8

YOUR SIXTIES
AND BEYOND

If you are in your sixties, seventies, or beyond, what you do now can be incredibly significant for how you age the rest of your life. Longevity is part of the motivation, but I've found that quality of life is even more important to my patients in this age range. How can you continue to improve your current and future well-being?

Exercise

Part of the answer is to focus on strength training and flexibility. You've got to move your body if you want to keep feeling great as you age. Strengthen and lengthen your muscles by making intentional movement part of your daily life. Going for a walk around the neighborhood is great, but you also need to get on the floor and stretch. There are countless flexibility programs you can find online, or you can work with a trainer who can teach you how to help protect yourself from injury by properly stretching specific muscles, tendons, and ligaments.

Cardiovascular exercise—getting your heart rate up for at least thirty minutes five days per week—is also mission critical in this season of life. This doesn't just improve your circulation and strengthen your heart, but it also has a positive impact on cognition and brain health. If your goal is to prevent cognitive decline and keep up with your grandkids, then cardio exercise needs to be in your routine. And be mindful that just because you aren't as interested in or capable of doing the same type or intensity of cardio you did when you were younger, there are still tons of ways you can be physically active. Riding bikes (outside or stationary), swimming, an elliptical trainer—those are all lower impact exercises that can still get your heart pumping and a good sweat going. Look for gyms that cater to your age range if that makes you more comfortable, or just turn on some good music and dance it out in your living room. Exercise should be fun.

Gut Health as You Age

The other part of improving your quality of life as you age has to do with gut health. Now, you've probably noticed I believe the topic of gut health is important in every decade of life. But I want to discuss it in-depth in this chapter, since this is the time when gastrointestinal (GI) symptoms can start to become an issue. They might manifest as polyps discovered on a colonoscopy, acid reflux, gallstones, fatty liver, stomach ulcers, or diverticulosis. If your gut is off, you can develop joint pain, stomach pain, weight gain, and autoimmune diseases, to name a few. Eating fiber, taking probiotics, limiting highly inflammatory foods like sugar, wheat, dairy, and alcohol can be very helpful. It's also important to avoid over-the-counter meds like ibuprofen as they can wreak havoc on the gut and cause long-term consequences like stomach ulcers and esophagitis.

The Connection Between Your Gut and Your Hormones

Your gut microbiome—which resides in your large intestine—is a huge piece of your body's hormone puzzle. In many ways, it's the starting point because if your gut is out of balance, it's impossible for your hormones or anything else to be in balance. In fact, you may have heard this before, but Hippocrates said more than two thousand years ago, "All disease begins in the gut." No matter how much you try to optimize other parts of your body, if your gut is out of balance, you will not be able to adequately attain the health you are seeking. And no matter how much you replace hormones in which you are deficient, you will not be optimized until you get your gut microbiome functioning properly.

While this is a rapidly developing area of research, it seems that issues within the gut could play a big role in the development of autoimmune diseases such as fibromyalgia, lupus, and Hashimoto's thyroiditis.[85] In fact, when a patient comes to me with an autoimmune diagnosis, one of the very first approaches to restoring their health is to evaluate their gut with a stool test and a breath test. This helps to evaluate for leaky gut, SIBO (small intestine bacterial overgrowth), inflammation, yeast overgrowth, parasites, and infection, and once these areas of the gut are healed, inflammation starts to decline. The majority of people who have been diagnosed with an autoimmune disease believe their only option is to manage it, usually with medications. Rarely do patients think they can reverse their autoimmune disease. But it's completely possible. The first step is often healing the gut.

What Is Your Gut Telling You?

I recently had a patient who came in to see me to address her menopausal concerns. After we discussed her symptoms, I asked her about her gut. She didn't really think much of it, but she explained to me that every time she ate, she had to run to the bathroom. She had accepted this as her normal for more than twenty years. She had talked to her doctor but nothing much seemed to help and she had just lived with it for all these years. When I told her that this was not normal and that we needed to fix it, she was relieved. When I told her that this was a reflection that her body was out of balance and it was causing other symptoms, she was surprised. So we analyzed her gut and sure enough, the bacteria in her gut were off and she had SIBO. I treated her and within a month, her IBS symptoms were gone. She couldn't believe it. She no longer was running to the bathroom every time she ate. She was finally able to enjoy a meal without looking for a restroom. It was a major shift in her quality of life.

The term "gut" gets thrown around a lot these days, but let's dig into this topic a bit more. You probably know that our bodies are host to trillions of microbes, including bacteria. Together, those microbes are referred to as *microbiota*, and the environment in which they live is the microbiome.[86] When we have just the right amounts of "good" microbes and not too many of the "bad" microbes, everything functions as it should. But when that balance is upset, and too many of the "bad" microbes begin to flourish, that's known as "gut dysbiosis." And the result of this dysbiosis can be a thinning of the intestinal lining, eventually leading to permeability.

When the gut lining has become permeable, we refer to that as leaky gut syndrome. A patient with leaky gut, or even just minor inflammation within the intestinal lining, might experience symptoms like bloating, painful gas, acid reflux, and other uncomfortable gastrointestinal symptoms. None of those symptoms are normal, and they should never be overlooked. They are often the first red flags your body is giving you that your balance is off, and the quicker you can address the real cause, the better. And I'm not just talking about masking those symptoms with over-the-counter medications that might provide temporary relief. In fact, many of those medications only serve to exacerbate the issue. Take a look at these red flag gut warnings and see if any apply to you.

Red Flag Warnings Your Gut Is Giving You

1. Acid reflux. If you often experience heartburn, don't just assume you have trouble digesting certain foods. Acid reflux is actually your body's way of telling you that the balance in your gut is off. Ironically, heartburn typically indicates that you are not producing enough stomach acid to

properly digest your food. And taking acid reflux medications, such as antacids, cause that imbalance to get even worse over time. That's why many antacid users find themselves needing more and more medication just to get through the day. And worse than that, you may have seen articles indicating that acid reflux medications are linked to dementia.[87] It is important to understand and uncover the underlying root cause of your heartburn, and not just continuously treat symptoms.

2. Constipation. In an ideal world, you should be having one to two bowel movements per day. They should be well-formed, and you should not have to strain to get them out. If you are not having a bowel movement every day, your gut is not working properly. Constipation is often the first sign that our gut balance is off and needs to be addressed. And keep in mind that stool is waste made up of bacteria, undigested food particles, and excess hormones. If you're not eliminating on a regular basis, that waste is just building up in your body. Treating constipation with laxatives is dangerous because extended use can actually cause your bowels to stop working properly on their own; and the use of laxatives can lead to

vitamin and mineral deficiencies, which in turn can create other health problems.

3. Irritable Bowel Syndrome (IBS). It's amazing how many patients I have seen over the years who suffer from irritable bowel syndrome. This is a cluster of symptoms that commonly includes diarrhea associated with food or stress but can also include bloating, abdominal pain, gas, and/ or constipation. If you regularly experience these symptoms, your body is not able to absorb food properly because the gut microbiome is not balanced. This could be due to an overgrowth of certain bacteria, fungi, or parasites. And as you know, the root cause must be treated. Anti-diarrheal medications are not the answer. Loperamide, for example, is an over-the-counter drug known as Imodium and can cause a range of side effects from dizziness to constipation, and even fast or irregular heartbeat and heart problems. Don't just think you can mask symptoms like diarrhea with over-the-counter medications; they all come with potential side effects.

4. Sugar cravings. This might not be the first thing you think of in terms of gut-related issues, but it's an important symptom to understand. Yeast

overgrowth (candida) or SIBO (small intestine bacterial overgrowth) can both cause you to crave sugar. With simple tests, a functional medicine physician can quickly discern if you have an overgrowth of bacteria in your small intestine (a topic we'll cover later in this chapter) or an overgrowth of candida. Sugar cravings can be resolved with dietary adjustments and specific supplements.*

5. Satiety issues. Do you ever get full soon after starting a meal? Or do you feel like you could eat all day long and never really feel satisfied? Both of those satiety issues tell you something about your gut. There are two main hormones involved in digesting food: ghrelin and leptin. Ghrelin is made in your stomach, and it sends hunger signals to your brain when you need to eat. Leptin lets you know when you've had enough food. If your gut balance is off, the production of these hormones can get disrupted. So, feeling too full or not full enough is another indicator that there's something worth investigating in your gut.

---

* For example, if you have SIBO, then there is a certain supplemental protocol for treating it that will reduce sugar cravings. You can check out www.siboinfo.com for more info on SIBO. Or if you have candida (yeast overgrowth), there are specific herbs that will reduce the yeast and in turn reduce the cravings. It's imperative that you get your gut tested to know the cause.

This list is really just scratching the surface, because the truth is, countless symptoms could point toward an imbalance in the gut. Skin irritations and other dermatological conditions; low-quality sleep; and emotional or mental health issues, including anxiety and depression, memory loss, and lack of focus, are all signs that your gut is unbalanced. So let's dive deeper into how we test for and identify what, specifically, is going on inside your gut, and how to heal it.

Functional Gut Diagnostic Testing

Doctors can discern so much about your gut function from a stool sample. I use a test by Genova Diagnostics called GI Effects. It provides a wealth of information about my patients' gut microbiome. It can detect dysbiosis and yeast, parasites, maldigestion, inflammation, and metabolite imbalance. Within each of those categories, it reveals exactly which microbiota your body has, and whether each is within a healthy range. This kind of specific diagnostic tool allows me to determine what kinds of foods my patient should be eating more or less of, which probiotics would be beneficial (and which ones to avoid), and much more. I highly recommend this test to almost everyone, even if you don't think you have any GI-related symptoms. As I've already covered, there are so many health issues that originate in the gut, and this test can help you and your doctor figure out what's going on in your body.

If SIBO is suspected, there is a breath test that can confirm it. SIBO is a common clinical condition characterized by excessive bacteria in the small intestine and can develop in a variety of patient populations. When bacteria not commonly found in the small intestine begin to flourish, a patient might experience chronic diarrhea, malnutrition, nausea, vomiting, unintentional weight loss, and more. You can conduct Genova's SIBO noninvasive breath test over two or three hours, right at home. Once you send your collection back to the lab, they will analyze the exhaled hydrogen and methane gases and determine if your small intestine is harboring an overgrowth of bacteria that do not belong there.

When considering gut health, a lot of people immediately assume they just need to start taking probiotics. This can actually make things worse. This is especially true if you do have SIBO because taking probiotics or eating fermented foods like sauerkraut, kimchi, kefir, or kombucha just feeds the overgrowth and can make your symptoms infinitely worse. It is best to have a full analysis of the bacterial makeup of your gut, which will show precisely what needs to be done in order to restore your gut health. When you have real data to work with, you know what steps to take, rather than just trying everything on the market that is labeled as "gut healthy" and then possibly harming your gut further.

How Hormones and Your Gut Fit Together

You might be wondering what the health of your gut has to do with your hormones and why I'm even covering it in this book. After all, if you've ever seen an endocrinologist about your thyroid or a gynecologist about your estrogen levels, it would be extremely rare if they ever initiated a discussion around the health of your gut microbiome. They treat the organ system they are trained to address and are not looking to treat your body as a whole. But as you probably realize by now, functional medicine takes the opposite approach; it considers the whole patient and understands that the body is synchronous and every system must be addressed in order to bring the entire body into homeostasis.

Did you know that the microbes in your gut are in constant communication with cells all over your body? The "gut-brain axis" refers to the complex communication networks among the gut, endocrine system, immune system, and autonomic nervous system. The bacteria and other microbes in your gut actually influence distant organs and pathways so much that gut microbiota is now considered to be a full-fledged endocrine organ.[88] The microbiota plays a major role in the reproductive endocrine system throughout a woman's lifetime by interacting with estrogen, androgen, insulin, and other hormones. Research even indicates that imbalances in the gut microbiota composition can lead to several diseases and conditions, such as pregnancy complications, polycystic ovarian syndrome (PCOS), endometriosis, and cancer.[89] This is an area of research that is rapidly evolving, but I've seen enough evidence just in my own practice to say with confidence that the origin of a vast array of health challenges, including hormonal imbalance, can be found within the gut.

Earlier I touched on the topic of estrogen dominance, which is an increased level of estrogen relative to the amount of progesterone that is found in the body. This condition can lead to debilitating issues including obesity, metabolic syndrome, cancer (including breast cancer), endometrial hyperplasia, endometriosis, polycystic ovarian syndrome, fertility, cardiovascular disease (CVD), and declining cognitive function.[90] An imbalance in the gut can actually lead to an imbalance in estrogen, causing hormones to recirculate. You are supposed to excrete excess estrogen, but when you are dealing with leaky gut, estrogen gets recirculated back into the system. That's how it begins to build up over time. But once you address the issues in your gut, your hormones often sort themselves out too. Your body is able to get back into a state of homeostasis and heal itself, if you give it the right tools.

Healing the Gut

Because healing your gut can lead to healing so many other ailments, I can't reiterate enough the importance of taking the steps discussed in this chapter. In fact, I want to share one patient's gut health journey to underscore this point:

I came to Dr. Taylor after losing all hope and reaching rock bottom. Amid many accomplishments as a business professional, father, and husband, the pressure of life started to affect my health, resulting in paralyzing panic attacks. Panic symptoms included nausea, diarrhea, lack of focus, dizziness, heart palpitations, and suicidal ideation. Nobody understood what was happening to me, and I always lived in a panicked state, afraid of the next attack to come. Over the next three years, I experimented with every kind of therapy: traditional talk therapy, hypnosis, EMDR, breath work, meditation, group therapy, and couple's therapy. I took two leaves of absence from work. I attended two in-patient programs, culminating in a nine month stay in a treatment facility, desperate to find anything that could curb my symptoms. And the prescription medications were the worst—going through about fifty different medications in three years created dependency, insomnia, and difficulty eating. I lost most of my relationships, and my marriage was severely strained. And then one day, my wife listened to a podcast about the health effects of inflammation; she suggested I find a functional medicine doctor. Dr. Taylor's name was the first name to come up on Google. Together, we tested my hormones and gut microbiome and discovered that I had been suffering from SIBO and leaky gut. I finally learned the connection between my gut and my brain. Simply clearing out gluten, dairy, sugar, and alcohol completely changed my life. These dietary changes, coupled with specific supplements prescribed by Dr. Taylor, created transformational change. I am forever grateful and indebted to Dr. Taylor and her entire practice. They got to the root cause of the issue while so many before had treated me as an "unfixable anomaly." It is my highest recommendation that you reach out to Dr. Taylor and take back control of your life!**

I am beyond grateful for the opportunity to assist patients like this in getting their lives back. I know there are so many people who feel like they've tried everything and exhausted all possibilities. Maybe you're one of them. My hope is that stories like this give you the confidence that treatment is available and you can bring your body back into balance. Healing the gut is not accomplished with a one-size-fits-all protocol. That's why testing is so essential—to provide data to determine the best course of action for your specific situation. But until you can get an appointment with a functional medicine doctor, you can get started on my gut health protocol. This isn't something

---

** Reprinted with permission of the patient.

you'll do forever; it's a temporary treatment that will help your gut begin the healing process.

Dr. Taylor's Gut Health Protocol

- Dietary changes:

  - No gluten (and limit gluten-free grains)

  - No dairy (this includes cheese, yogurt, cream, milk, ice cream, and any other products made with dairy)

  - No alcohol

  - No caffeine (this includes coffee, caffeinated sparkling drinks, soda, caffeinated teas, etc.)

  - No refined sugar (become a label reader—there's added sugar in many foods you wouldn't expect)

  - No diet drinks. Artificial sweeteners are toxic.

  - Aim for an anti-inflammatory diet that includes plenty of cruciferous vegetables (broccoli, cauliflower, etc.), healthy fats like avocado and coconut oil, and nutrient-dense fish.

- Avoid seed oils.

- Limit meats, and when you do eat meat, ensure it is organic and lean.

- Avoid processed foods. Avoid packaged and canned foods as much as possible. Instead, shop the perimeter of the grocery store, focusing on fresh, whole foods like produce, grass-fed animal meat, free-range eggs, fresh organic herbs, etc.

- Supplements: Be intentional about the vitamins and supplements you take, as some of them can negatively impact GI symptoms.*** Make sure everything you take is very high quality (which is tough to navigate on your own, and a doctor or nutritionist can give you a lot more insight into which supplements are high quality and which ones are not), and that you are only taking supplements that are appropriate for you *based on testing.* (Tip: Don't just willy-nilly order some supplements off an Instagram link.)

  - I know it's tempting when you hear about

*** For instance, probiotics can give you worse GI symptoms if you have undiagnosed SIBO, and some additives in some vitamins can cause bloating, gas, or diarrhea.

some new "fad" supplement, but supplements should be individualized and patient-specific. Until you get your GI test results, avoid taking broad-spectrum probiotics.

Your gut plays a significant role in your overall health, wellness, and hormonal balance. Knowledge is power, so I encourage you to work with your functional medicine physician to test' your gut microbiome and then use that data to heal your gut. You'll be so glad you did.

Dr. Taylor's Sixties-and-Beyond Checklist

- Estrogen balance is important for women to decrease the risk of cardiovascular disease, protect the bones, and protect the brain from dementia.

- Testosterone helps to build bone mass and is important for preventing osteoporosis.

- Avoid over-the-counter medication like Tylenol, which can damage your liver, and NSAIDs, which can damage your stomach.

- Take turmeric for inflammation. (Discuss brands and quantities with your practitioner.)

- Get your gut microbiome and digestion in order. Do a comprehensive stool and breath test yearly.

- Get quality sleep. It helps to reset everything.

- Stay hydrated. Your kidneys depend on it.

- Take a supplement for your brain health. Omegas and gingko biloba are both good to take daily.

- Take a good antioxidant like glutathione or NAC. This is important for detoxifying so that your liver can then properly metabolize your hormones.

- Avoid medication if at all possible.

- Have a really good PCP (primary care physician) and a really good functional medicine physician. This is a great combination as you age.

- Stay busy and active.

Chapter 9

YOUR GUIDE TO FINDING A FUNCTIONAL MEDICINE PHYSICIAN

I love functional medicine and I think everyone should have a functional medicine physician in their corner, regardless of age. As I shared with you earlier, I had never even *heard* of functional medicine in my early med school days; it just wasn't talked about. So I had to figure it all out on my own. But I don't want you to have to figure it out on your own, so let's talk about how you can take advantage of this wonderful field of medicine.

The Institute for Functional Medicine is a great resource for training medical doctors to practice functional medicine. The institute provides critical information to doctors so they can understand how to look at every patient as a whole, rather than just zero in on chasing symptoms. As you know by this point in the book, much of what I practice is based on hormones, and this has a profoundly positive impact on my patients. However, hormones are not the whole picture. The body is integrated, and all systems are connected, so treating the whole body is key.

Functional medicine identifies and addresses the root cause of disease. So if a patient's hormones are imbalanced, a functional medicine doctor approaches the problem by becoming a "detective" to discover why. But you're probably wondering how you can find a doctor who can do all of this and really become a partner in improving your health. I suggest starting at the Institute for Functional Medicine's website (www.ifm.org), where you can click "Find a Practitioner," and thus begin your search for someone near you. I'm also working to expand my reach via my telemedicine platform, so you can always check out my website at www.julietaylormd.com to find out more. I also love pointing people in the right direction to receive the gold standard in medical care, so don't hesitate to reach out to me via my website. I'd be happy to hear from you.

Again, I really believe *everyone* should have a functional medicine physician, no matter where you are on the spectrum of age and current health status. Currently my youngest patient is four years old and comes to see me for gut healing after several rounds of antibiotics. My oldest patient is ninety-five years old and comes to see me for a testosterone boost so he can continue his daily hikes in the local mountains. So it's never too early or too late to start. Whether you're a teenager dealing with the first signs of PMS, a woman in her thirties battling postpartum symptoms, or a sixty-something-year-old wishing she had more energy to engage with her family, functional medicine can help you. Looking at and treating the root cause of imbalances or illnesses is so much more effective and logical than simply treating symptoms.

I know cost can be a challenge. As of the writing of this book, insurance does not typically cover functional medicine. But the more people are aware of this type of practice and advocate for coverage, the closer we will get to insurance companies recognizing this as an essential part of the health-care system. It leads to healthier, more vibrant individuals who can contribute to their families, communities, and society. Plus, it's important to think about the expense as an investment in your health and your future. Paying a little more now for top-notch care and guidance will help you resolve health issues before they become full-fledged illness. And *that* can save you a lot of money, pain, and heartache in the future. I hope you'll start your search today for a functional medicine practitioner to come alongside you.

CONCLUSION

If I had to choose one main message that I want you to glean from this book, it's this: Think outside of the box when it comes to your health. Just because your doctor says everything is within normal range, look further for an answer. Find someone who will sit and listen to you and do the right tests to solve the problem. Your health is ultimately in your hands, and you have the ability to navigate your way toward optimal wellness. I hope this book provides a tool to be able to navigate your health in a way that is meaningful and productive.

As I said in the author's note, though we are all unique and each of us is on our own journey, there are some universal truths that apply to everyone. What I've aimed to do within these pages is to give you the beginnings of a manual, one that you can use to bring your hormones back into balance. It's hard to be at your best if you're simply not feeling great. Once you understand and know that you have options, however, you will believe that you *can* feel great. I think you'll very quickly discover that using this book as your guide will get you from believing to actually seeing results.

Whenever I start thinking and talking about women's health in general, I find myself feeling disappointed in the American medical system. It is not geared toward empowering women to live their best lives. Recently, I was floored when a patient came to me and said that her general physician was concerned about the hormone pellets I'd prescribed to her and wanted her to quit using them. When she asked what he proposed to do for treating her symptoms, should they return after stopping hormones, he suggested a different prescription pill for each of her symptoms. There was one pill for her depression, another pill for her sleep, and another for her joint pain. Those had all been relieved with balancing her hormones. This is just one example of a doctor beholden to a broken system and a "standard of care" that prefers Band-Aid solutions rather than treating the root cause of the issue. (Needless to say, my patient opted to stick with the pellets.)

I especially feel frustrated when it comes to how the American medical system generally treats postpartum mothers. I covered it in this book, but I still have much to say on the topic, so I'm sure you'll hear a lot more from me. I am an advocate for mothers, and I want all moms to hear this message: postpartum depression should not be tolerated. It is a sign of hormone imbalance, and it needs to be treated by addressing and fixing hormones.

I really, truly hope you use this book as a tool, as a manual for your hormones. Give it to your sister, your best friend, your mother, your daughter. Give it to your neighbor who just had a baby. Give it to your coworker who is going through menopause. The more we learn, the more we can teach others, and the better we understand ourselves, the more we will get the treatment we need when things don't seem right. Getting to the root of the problem is key. Be hopeful, be your best advocate, and be well!

XO

ACKNOWLEDGMENTS

This book would not exist without the steadfast support and collaborative efforts of so many remarkable individuals. First, I want to extend my deepest gratitude to Lisa Clark, who believed in this project from its earliest stages. Her extraordinary ability to capture my vision and bring it to life on the page has been nothing short of transformative.

I am equally thankful for the talented team at Forefront Books. Becky Nesbitt, my publisher, offered unwavering support and guidance that kept me energized throughout the writing and editing process. Jill Smith, Sr. Editor, oversaw every detail, guaranteeing that the final product was even better than I could have imagined. My heartfelt thanks go out to the rest of the Forefront team for their dedication and expertise.

I also want to honor my educational roots at Michigan State University and Loma Linda

University. To all the professors who challenged me, encouraged me, and helped shape my approach to medicine—thank you for your guidance and dedication. I am equally grateful to the institutions and educational programs I've studied under, which champion a holistic approach to healthcare and train MDs to practice functional medicine. A heartfelt thanks goes out to the many MDs who have gone before me, whose pioneering work continues to pave the way for future functional medicine leaders.

Finally, I must acknowledge my wonderful family. Their unwavering encouragement and the precious time and space they afforded me to research, write, and refine these pages made all the difference. My love and admiration for you is endless. And of course, my mom and dad. You are my backbone; you are unwavering and unconditional in your love and support and I love you both beyond words.

No project is ever finished in isolation—this book stands as a testament that with the support of an incredible team, dreams truly become reality.

To everyone who contributed to this journey, thank you for believing in *The Hormone Manual* and for helping transform a simple idea into a guide that I hope will empower women at every stage of life.

NOTES

1. Rossouw JE, Anderson GL, Prentice RL, LaCroix AZ, Kooperberg C, Stefanick ML, Jackson RD, Beresford SA, Howard BV, Johnson KC, Kotchen JM, Ockene J; Writing Group for the Women's Health Initiative Investigators. Risks and benefits of estrogen plus progestin in healthy postmenopausal women: principal results From the Women's Health Initiative randomized controlled trial. JAMA. 2002 Jul 17; 288 (3):321-33. doi: 10.1001/jama.288.3.321. PMID: 12117397.

2. D. W. Sturdee et al., "Updated IMS Recommendations on Postmenopausal Hormone Therapy and Preventive Strategies for Midlife Health," *Climacteric* 14, no. 3 (2011): 302–20, https://doi.org/10.3109/136971 37.2011.570590.

3. Avrum Bluming, Howard Hodis, and Robert Langer, "'Tis but a Scratch: A Critical Review of the Women's Health Initiative Evidence Associating Menopausal Hormone Therapy with the Risk of Breast Cancer," *Menopause* 30, no. 12 (December 2023): 1241–45, https://doi.org/10.1097/GME.0000000000002267.

4. David S. Meyers et al., "Primary Care Physicians' Perceptions of the Effect of Insurance Status on Clinical Decision Making," *Annals of Family Medicine* 4, no. 5 (2006): 399-402, https://doi.org/10.1370/afm.574.

5. Chelsea Moore et al., "Integrating Cultural Humility Into Infant Safe Sleep Counseling: A Pediatric Resident Simulation," *Cureus* 13, no. 12 (December 31, 2021): e20847, https://doi.org/10.7759/cureus.20847.

6. Chitaru Tokutake et al., "Infant Suffocation Incidents Related to Co-Sleeping or Breastfeeding in the Side-Lying Position in Japan," *The Tohoku Journal of Experimental Medicine* 246, no. 2 (2018): 121-130, released on J-STAGE October 24, 2018, https://doi.org/10.1620/tjem.246.121, https://www.jstage.jst.go.jp/article/tjem/246/2/246_121/_article/-char/en.

7. Tasuku Okui, "Association Between Infant Mortality and Parental Educational Level: An Analysis of Data from Vital Statistics and Census in Japan," *PLOS ONE* 18, no. 6 (June 14, 2023): e0286530, https://doi.org/10.1371/journal.pone.0286530.

8. National Center for Health Statistics, Centers for Disease Control and Prevention, "Provisional Life Expectancy Estimates for 2021," accessed July 22, 2024. https://www.cdc.gov/nchs/data/vsrr/vsrr033.pdf.

9. Mandy Major, "What Postpartum Care Looks Like Around the World, and Why the U.S. Is Missing the Mark," Healthline, March 26, 2020, https://www.healthline.com/health/pregnancy/what-post-childbirth-care-looks-like-around-the-world-and-why-the-u-s-is-missing-the-mark.

10. Christopher J. Stewart et al., "Temporal Development of the Gut Microbiome in Early Childhood from the TEDDY Study," Nature 562 (2018): 583–88, https://doi.org/10.1038/s41586-018-0617-x.

11. Maria Mousikou, Andreas Kyriakou, and Nicos Skordis, "Stress and Growth in Children and Adolescents," Hormone Research in Paediatrics 96, no. 1 (2023): 25–33, https://doi.org/10.1159/000521074.

12. M. P. Francino, "Antibiotics and the Human Gut Microbiome: Dysbioses and Accumulation of Resistances," Frontiers in Microbiology 6 (January 12, 2016): 1543, https://doi.org/10.3389/fmicb.2015.01543.

13. Walaa K. Mousa et al., "Microbial Dysbiosis in the Gut Drives Systemic Autoimmune Diseases," *Frontiers in Immunology* 13 (October 20, 2022): 906258, https://doi.org/10.3389/fimmu.2022.906258.

14. Michael J. Panza et al., "Adolescent Sport Participation and Symptoms of Anxiety and Depression: A Systematic Review and Meta-Analysis," Journal of Sport and Exercise Psychology 42, no. 3 (May 2020): 201–18, https://doi.org/10.1123/jsep.2019-0235.

15. Jean M. Twenge, Garrett C. Hisler, and Zlatan Krizan, "Associations Between Screen Time and Sleep Duration Are Primarily Driven by Portable Electronic Devices: Evidence from a Population-Based Study of U.S. Children Ages 0–17," Sleep Medicine 56 (April 2019): 211–18, https://doi.org/10.1016/j.sleep.2018.11.009.

16. Lauren Hale and Stanford Guan, "Screen Time and Sleep Among School-Aged Children and Adolescents: A Systematic Literature Review," Sleep Medicine Reviews 21 (June 2015): 50–8, https://doi.org/10.1016/j.smrv.2014.07.007.

17. Xiaojie Sun et al., "Associations of Glyphosate Exposure and Serum Sex Steroid Hormones Among 6–19-Year-Old Children and Adolescents," Ecotoxicology and Environmental Safety 275 (2024): 116266, https://doi.org/10.1016/j.ecoenv.2024.116266.

18. Marcelino Pérez-Bermejo et al., "The Role of Bisphenol A in Diabetes and Obesity," Biomedicines 9, no. 6 (June 10, 2021): 666, https://doi.org/10.3390/biomedicines9060666.

19. Charlotte Skovlund et al., "Association of Hormonal Contraception with Depression," JAMA Psychiatry 73, no. 11 (2016): 1154–62, https://doi.org/10.1001/jamapsychiatry.2016.2387.

20. Shilpi Rajoria et al., "3,3'-Diindolylmethane Modulates Estrogen Metabolism in Patients with Thyroid Proliferative Disease: A Pilot Study," Thyroid 21, no. 3 (2011): 299–304, https://doi.org/10.1089/thy.2010.0245.

21. Sylvia Kiconco et al., "Menstrual Cycle Regularity as a Predictor for Heart Disease and Diabetes: Findings from a Large Population-Based Longitudinal Cohort Study," Clinical Endocrinology 96, no. 4 (2022): 605–616, https://doi.org/10.1111/cen.14640.

22. Yi-Xin Wang et al., "Menstrual Cycle Regularity and Length across the Reproductive Lifespan and Risk of Premature Mortality: Prospective Cohort Study," BMJ 371 (2020): m3464, https://doi.org/10.1136/bmj.m3464.

23. Cirillo et al., "Irregular Menses Predicts Ovarian Cancer: Prospective Evidence from the Child Health and Development Studies," International Journal of Cancer 139, no. 5 (2016):1009–17, https://doi.org/10.1002/ijc.30144.

24. Walaa K. Mousa et al., "Microbial Dysbiosis in the Gut Drives Systemic Autoimmune Diseases," *Frontiers in Immunology* 13 (October 20, 2022): 906258, https://doi.org/10.3389/fimmu.2022.906258.

25. Malik, T. F., and K. K. Panuganti, "Lactose Intolerance," In *StatPearls* [Internet], updated April 17, 2023, Treasure Island, FL: StatPearls Publishing, January 2024-. Available from https://www.ncbi.nlm.nih.gov/books/NBK532285/.

26. Forks Over Knives, directed by Lee Fulkerson, Virgil Films, 2011.

27. "Newsletter #2 (Winter 1991): Seventy-Fifth Anniversary of the Brownsville Clinic," The Margaret Sanger Papers Project, accessed June 29, 2024, https://sanger.hosting.nyu.edu/articles/seventieth_anniversary_of_brownsville/.

28. Theresa Vargas, "Guinea Pigs or Pioneers? How Puerto Rican Women Were Used to Test the Birth Control Pill," Washington Post, May 9, 2017, https://www.washingtonpost.com/news/retropolis/wp/2017/05/09/guinea-pigs-or-pioneers-how-puerto-rican-women-were-used-to-test-the-birth-control-pill/.

29. "The Pill in America," American Experience, PBS, accessed June 29, 2024, https://www.pbs.org/wgbh/americanexperience/features/pill-america/.

30. Annette Fuentes, "Books on Health: Birth Control from 'Womb Veils' to Lysol," New York Times, June 12, 2001, https://www.nytimes.com/2001/06/12/health/books-on-health-birth-control-from-womb-veils-to-lysol.html.

31. "Pill Senate Holds Hearings on the Pill, 1970," American Experience, PBS, accessed July 22, 2024, https://www.pbs.org/wgbh/americanexperience/features/pill-senate-holds-hearings-pill-1970/.

32. Kristin Compton, "Yaz Settlements," Drugwatch, last modified September 5, 2023, https://www.drugwatch.com/yaz/settlements.

33. "Brown Requires Bayer to Launch $20 Million Ad Campaign to Correct," State of California Department of Justice—Office of the Attorney General, February 9, 2009, https://oag.ca.gov/news/press-releases/brown-requires-bayer-launch-20-million-ad-campaign-correct-misleading.

34. "Seasonique and Seasonale Lawsuit Filed, Claiming Birth Control Pills Caused Liver Tumors," AboutLawsuits.com, June 6, 2017, https://www.aboutlawsuits.com/seasonique-and-seasonale-lawsuit-128975/.

35. "First Over-the-Counter Daily Contraceptive Pill Released," American College of Obstetricians and Gynecologists, March 2024, https://www.acog.org/clinical/clinical-guidance/practice-advisory/articles/2024/03/first-over-the-counter-daily-contraceptive-pill-released.

36. "Opill (0.075 mg Oral Norgestrel Tablet) Information," U.S. Food and Drug Administration, accessed July 22, 2024, https://www.fda.gov/drugs/postmarket-drug-safety-information-patients-and-providers/opill-0075mg-oral-norgestrel-tablet-information#:~:text=Common%20side%20effects%20may%20include,important%20to%20seek%20medical%20advice.

37. Writing Group for the Women's Health Initiative Investigators, "Risks and Benefits of Estrogen Plus Progestin in Healthy Postmenopausal Women: Principal Results From the Women's Health Initiative Randomized Controlled Trial," JAMA 288, no. 3 (2002): 321-333, https://doi.org/10.1001/jama.288.3.321.

38. "Infertility FAQs," Centers for Disease Control and Prevention, accessed July 22, 2024, https://www.cdc.gov/reproductive-health/infertility-faq/.

39. "IVF-Assisted Pregnancies Constitute 2% of All Babies Born in the United States in 2022." American Society for Reproductive Medicine. Accessed July 22, 2024. https://www.asrm.org/news-and-events/asrm-news/press-releasesbulletins/ivf-assisted-pregnancies-constitute/#:~:text=In%202022%2C%20the%20number%20of,result%20of%20successful%20ART%20cycles.

40. "Forbes Health: How Much Does IVF Cost?" Forbes, accessed July 22, 2024, https://www.forbes.com/health/womens-health/how-much-does-ivf-cost/.

41. "Clinic Summary Report: Multiple Year Comparison," Society for Assisted Reproductive Technology, accessed July 22, 2024, https://www

.sartcorsonline.com/rptCSR_PublicMultYear.aspx?ClinicPKID=0 #patient-first-attempt.

42. Mikkelsen et al., 2013, "Pre-Gravid Oral Contraceptive Use and Time to Pregnancy: A Danish Prospective Cohort Study," Human Reproduction 28 (5): 1398–1405. https://doi.org/10.1093/humrep/det023.

43. Ellen M. Mikkelsen et al., "Pre-Gravid Oral Contraceptive Use and Time to Pregnancy: A Danish Prospective Cohort Study," Human Reproduction 28, no. 5 (2013): 1398–1405, https://doi.org/10.1093/humrep/det023.

44. "Long-Term Oral Contraceptive Use Doesn't Hurt Fertility, Study Finds," Boston University School of Public health, April 4, 2013, https://www.bu.edu/sph/news/articles/2013/long-term-oral-contraceptive-use-doesnt-hurt-fertility-study-finds/.

45. Nayana Talukdar, "Effect of Long-Term Combined Oral Contraceptive Pill Use on Endometrial Thickness," Obstetrics and Gynecology 120, no. 2 (part 1) (August 2012): 348–54, https://doi.org/10.1097/AOG.0b013e31825ec2ee.

46. C. C. Standley, "Birth Control Technology: Today and Tomorrow," Draper Fund Report (October 1980): 23–5, https://pubmed.ncbi.nlm.nih.gov/12310011/.

47. Kimberly Daniels and Joyce C. Abma, "Current Contraceptive Status Among Women Aged 15–49: United States, 2015–2017," NCHS Data Brief no. 327, CDC—National Center for Health Statistics, December 2018, https://www.cdc.gov/nchs/products/databriefs/db327.htm.

48. Ke Xun Chen et al., "Oral Contraceptive Use is Associated with Smaller Hypothalamic and Pituitary Gland Volumes in Healthy Women: A Structural MRI Study," PloS One 16, no. 4 (2021): e0249482, https://doi.org/10.1371/journal.pone.0249482.

49. Fleischman, Diana S., C. David Navarrete, and Daniel M.T. Fessler, "Oral Contraceptives Suppress Ovarian Hormone Production." Psychological Science 21, no. 5 (n.d.): 750–752. https://doi.org/10.1177/0956797610368062.

50. Bataa, Munkhtuya et al., "Exploring Progesterone Deficiency in First-Trimester Miscarriage and the Impact of Hormone Therapy on Foetal Development: A Scoping Review," Children (Basel, Switzerland) vol. 11,4 422, 2 Apr. 2024, doi:10.3390/children11040422.

51. Benson, Lyndsey S et al., "Early Pregnancy Loss Management in the Emergency Department vs Outpatient Setting," JAMA network open vol. 6,3 e232639, 1 Mar. 2023, doi:10.1001/jamanetworkopen.2023.2639.

52. Mughal, Saba, Yusra Azhar, and Waquar Siddiqui, "Postpartum Depression," StatPearls - NCBI Bookshelf. Last modified October 7, 2022, https://www.ncbi.nlm.nih.gov/books/NBK519070/.

53. S. Mughal, Y. Azhar, and W. Siddiqui, "Postpartum Depression," last updated October 7, 2022, in StatPearls [Internet] (Treasure Island, FL: StatPearls Publishing, January 2024), https://www.ncbi.nlm.nih.gov/books/NBK519070/.

54. "Perinatal Depression," US Department of Health and Human Services, National Institute of Mental Health, 2023, https://www.nimh.nih.gov/health/publications/perinatal-depression.

55. Mary Caffrey, "Obstetricians Are Well-Positioned to Diagnose, Treat Postpartum Depression, Speakers Say," American Journal of Managed Care, April 28, 2018, https://www.ajmc.com/view/obstetricians-are-well-positioned-to-diagnose-treat-postpartum-depression-speakers-say.

56. Medical Tests: Serum Progesterone," UCSF Health, April 1, 2023, https://www.ucsfhealth.org/medical-tests/serum-progesterone.

57. Robert Winston and Rebecca Chicot, "The Importance of Early Bonding on the Long-Term Mental Health and Resilience of Children," London Journal of Primary Care (Abingdon) 8, no. 1 (February 2016): 12–14, https://doi.org/10.1080/17571472.2015.1133012.

58. Adams, Rebecca, "How America Got Family Leave—And How It Failed," The Atlantic, last modified November 22, 2021, https://www.theatlantic.com/family/archive/2021/11/us-paid-family-parental-leave-congress-bill/620660/.

59. "FDA Approves First Treatment for Postpartum Depression," US Food and Drug Administration, March 19, 2019, from https://www.fda.gov/news-events/press-announcements/fda-approves-first-treatment-postpartum-depression.

60. "Brexanolone (Intravenous Route)," last modified February 11, 2024, https://www.mayoclinic.org/drugs-supplements/brexanolone-intravenous-route/proper-use/drg-20458449.

61. "Brexanolone (Intravenous Route)," last modified February 11, 2024, https://www.mayoclinic.org/drugs-supplements/brexanolone-intravenous-route/precautions/drg-20458449.

62. U.S. Food and Drug Administration. "FDA Approves First Oral Treatment for Postpartum Depression," Press Announcements, August 4, 2023, https://www.fda.gov/news-events/press-announcements/fda-approves-first-oral-treatment-postpartum-depression.

63. Narvaez, Darcia, "How Co-Sleeping Can Help You and Your Baby," Greater Good Magazine, October 14, 2018. https://greatergood.berkeley.edu/article/item/how_cosleeping_can_help_you_and_your_baby.

64. Ibid.

65. Wendy Middlemiss et al., "Asynchrony of Mother-Infant Hypothalam-

ic-Pituitary-Adrenal Axis Activity Following Extinction of Infant Crying Responses Induced During the Transition to Sleep," Early Human Development 88, no. 4 (April 2012): 227–232, https://doi.org/10.1016/j.earlhumdev.2011.08.010; Martin Reite, ed., The Psychobiology of Attachment and Separation (Academic Press, 2012).

66. Isnaini Herawati et al., "Breathing Exercise for Hypertensive Patients: A Scoping Review," Frontiers in Physiology 14 (January 2023), https://doi.org/10.3389/fphys.2023.1048338.

67. Yifei Zhang et al., "Treatment of Type 2 Diabetes and Dyslipidemia with the Natural Plant Alkaloid Berberine," Journal of Clinical Endocrinology & Metabolism 93, no. 7 (July 2008): 2559–65, https://doi.org/10.1210/jc.2007-2404.

68. Susan R. Davis and Glenn D. Braunstein, "Efficacy and Safety of Testosterone in the Management of Hypoactive Sexual Desire Disorder in Postmenopausal Women," Journal of Sexual Medicine 9, no. 4 (April 2012): 1134–48, https://doi.org/10.1111/j.1743-6109.2011.02634.x.

69. Chiara Achilli et al., "Efficacy and Safety of Transdermal Testosterone in Postmenopausal Women with Hypoactive Sexual Desire Disorder: A Systematic Review and Meta-Analysis," Fertility and Sterility 107, no. 2 (2017): 475–482, https://doi.org/10.1016/j.fertnstert.2016.10.028.

70. Gary S. Donovitz, "A Personal Prospective on Testosterone Therapy in Women—What We Know in 2022," *Journal of Personalized Medicine* 12, no. 8 (July 2022): 1194, https://doi.org/10.3390/jpm12081194.

71. M. F. Sowers et al., "Testosterone Concentrations in Women Aged 25–50 Years: Associations with Lifestyle, Body Composition, and Ovarian Status," American Journal of Epidemiology 153, no. 3 (February 2001): 256–64, https://doi.org/10.1093/aje/153.3.256.

72. Rebecca Glaser and Constantine Dimitrakakis, "Testosterone Therapy in Women: Myths and Misconceptions," Maturitas 74, no. 3 (March 2013): 230–34, https://doi.org/10.1016/j.maturitas.2013.01.003.

73. Ibid.

74. Glaser, Rebecca, Anne E York, and Constantine Dimitrakakis, "Beneficial Effects of Testosterone Therapy in Women Measured by the Validated Menopause Rating Scale (MRS)," Maturitas 68, no. 4 (April 1, 2011): 355–361. https://doi.org/10.1016/j.maturitas.2010.12.001.

75. Ibid.

76. Ibid.

77. Ibid.

78. Abhirami Ratnakumar et al., "Estrogen Activates Alzheimer's Disease Genes," Alzheimer's & Dementia: Translational Research & Clinical Interventions 5, no. 1 (2019): 906–17, https://doi.org/10.1016/j.trci.2019.09.004; James W. Simpkins et al., "The Potential for Estrogens

in Preventing Alzheimer's Disease and Vascular Dementia," Therapeutic
Advances in Neurological Disorders 2, no. 1 (January 2009): 31–49.

79. "More than Half of U.S. Adults Don't Know Heart Disease Is Leading
     Cause of Death, despite 100-Year Reign," American Heart Association,
     https://newsroom.heart.org/news/more-than-half-of-u-s-adults-dont-
     know-heart-disease-is-leading-cause-of-death-despite-100-year-reign.

80. "Estrogen Therapy in Early Menopause May Help Keep Arteries Clear,"
     American Heart Association News, March 3, 2020, https://www.heart
     .org/en/news/2020/03/03/estrogen-therapy-in-early-menopause-may-
     help-keep-arteries-clear.

81. F. Gersh, J. H. O'Keefe, A. Elagizi, C. J. Lavie, and J. A. Laukkanen,
     "Estrogen and Cardiovascular Disease," *Progress in Cardiovascular Diseases*
     84 (2024): 60–66.

82. Rebecca Glaser and Constantine Dimitrakakis, "Testosterone Therapy
     in Women: Myths and Misconceptions," Maturitas 74, no. 3 (March
     2013): 230–34, https://doi.org/10.1016/j.maturitas.2013.01.003.

83. Andre Guay and Susan R. Davis, "Testosterone Insufficiency in
     Women: Fact or fiction?" World Journal of Urology 20 (2002):106–10,
     https://doi.org10.1007/s00345-002-0267-2.

84. Manson, JoAnn E et al., "Menopausal hormone therapy and health
     outcomes during the intervention and extended poststopping phases of
     the Women's Health Initiative randomized trials," JAMA vol. 310,13
     (2013): 1353-68. doi:10.1001/jama.2013.278040.

85. Walaa Abdelaty Shaheen, Mohammed Nabil Quraishi, Tariq H Iqbal,
     Gut microbiome and autoimmune disorders, Clinical and Experimen-
     tal Immunology, Volume 209, Issue 2, August 2022, pages 161–174,
     https://doi.org/10.1093/cei/uxac057.

86. Markus MacGill, "What Are the Gut Microbiota and Human Microbi-
     ome?" Medical News Today, updated February 15, 2023, https://www.
     medicalnewstoday.com/articles/307998.

87. "Another Study Links PPIs and Dementia: AGA Expert Weighs In,"
     American Gastroenterological Association, August 9, 2023, https://gas-
     tro.org/news/study-links-long-term-ppi-use-with-dementia/.

88. Gerard Clarke et al., "Minireview: Gut Microbiota: The Neglect-
     ed Endocrine Organ," Molecular Endocrinology 28, no. 8 (August
     2014):1221–38, https://doi.org/10.1210/me.2014-1108.

89. Xinyu Qi et al., "The Impact of the Gut Microbiota on the Reproductive
     and Metabolic Endocrine System," Gut Microbes 13, no. 1 (Jan–Dec
     2021):1–21, https://doi.org/10.1080/19490976.2021.1894070.

90. James M. Baker et al., "Estrogen-Gut Microbiome Axis: Physiological
     and Clinical Implications," Maturitas 103 (September 2017): 45–53,
     https://doi.org/10.1016/j.maturitas.2017.06.025.

ABOUT THE AUTHOR

D r. Julie Taylor is a bioidentical hormone specialist and functional medicine doctor, with a thriving practice in Pasadena, California. She aims to restore health and wellness to her patients by treating the whole person. She sees patients—men and women of all ages—in her practice, where she emphasizes preventive medicine, reversing chronic disease, and finding the root cause of all symptoms. She focuses especially on menopause management and helping women find quality of life as they age. Born and raised in the Los Angeles area, Dr. Taylor received her medical degree from Michigan State University. She earned her master's in public health and completed residency training in preventive medicine at Loma Linda University. In 2014, upon finishing residency, she started her medical practice.

Dr. Taylor prides herself on being an

excellent clinician and finding connections with all her patients. But her first joy—what drives her more than anything—is her family. She and her husband, Drew, met while she was studying medicine and he was studying law in Michigan. They have three very active children. As a family, they enjoy spending time together traveling, hiking, skiing, and attending the kids' many sports games.

For more life-changing information,
go to www.JulieTaylorMD.com